The Complete Guide To Sandbag Training

Images by Alison Crocker

First Edition

For more information visit www.sandbagfitness.blogspot.com

Contents

Chapters	Page
Disclaimer	5
Foreword	5
Introduction	6
What Is Sandbag Fitness?	7
The Benefits of Sandbag Training	9
Equipment	13
How To Make This Programme Work	19
How To Grip The Sandbag	21
Warm ups	23
The Exercises	26
Squat & Lunge	27
Deadlift	40
Press/Push	43
Pull	54
Core	66
Full Body	79
Programmes	89
Beginner Programme	92
Intermediate Programme	120
Advanced Programme	148
FAQ	177
Connect With Us	181
Glossary	182

Disclaimer

The Complete Guide To Sandbag Training is not meant to diagnose or treat any medical condition. It is designed as a resource for individuals wishing to follow a progressive strength and conditioning programme using sandbags. Individuals with any pre-existing medical conditions should check with their doctor/physician before commencing any programme of physical activity.

I cannot be held responsible for any injury or medical complication resulting from the use or mis-use of this guide or any of the information contain herein.

If you are unsure about it's suitability for you, always check with a medical professional first.

Foreword

Welcome to the revised and expanded Complete Guide To Sandbag Training. This new edition contains a fully updated exercise section alongside three 10-week programmes for Beginner, Intermediate and Advanced.

Since releasing the 68-page Sandbag Fitness Training Manual in 2011, Sandbag Fitness and the sandbag lifting community has continued to grow at an impressive rate. It continues to be a source of passion for me - helping others to improve their health and fitness in such a simple way is, in this day and age, very important. Sandbag Fitness is still a no-nonsense, tough training regime and that isn't set to change anytime soon.

One of the major points of feedback after the Sandbag Fitness Manual was that people wanted more advanced exercises and training programmes. The Complete Guide To Sandbag Training contains just that. But, as always, results come from a progressive approach to exercise and I continue to get the best results from focusing on the basics. I urge you to do the same.

I hope you get as much enjoyment from this guide as I did writing it.

Train Hard!
Matt, Sandbag Fitness

Introduction

Welcome to the Complete Guide To Sandbag Training - a resource designed to allow you to train effectively from home with sandbags. This training guide contains detailed instructions of all that you need to build your own strength and conditioning programme.

I started the Sandbag Fitness Blog as a record of the training that I was doing in my garage - 2 years on and there is now a growing community of sandbag trainees.

Learn the exercises, follow the programmes and take part in the weekly workouts on the Sandbag Fitness Blog.

This manual is a detailed breakdown of the things I do to stay fit - with no omissions, propaganda or marketing spin. The training is tough but I think the results are worth it.

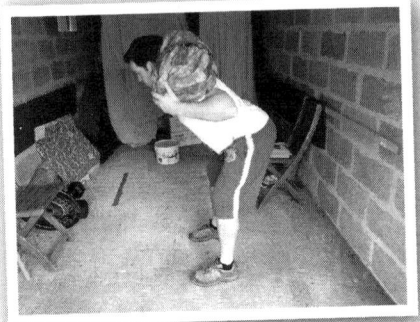

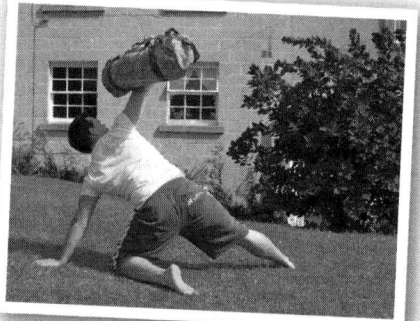

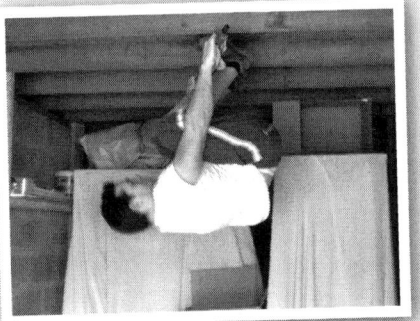

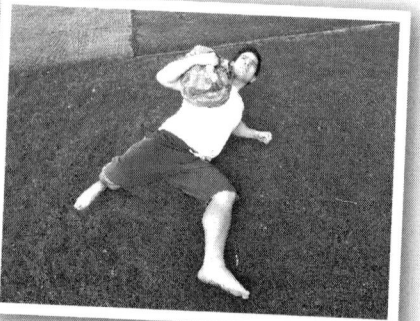

What Is Sandbag Fitness?

The concept behind Sandbag Fitness is simple - we help people to get fit using sandbags. I developed it as a resource for individuals who wanted to stay fit and incorporate sandbag training into their exercise regime. It's particularly useful for the following people:

- Those who cannot afford a gym membership or the cost of regular classes
- Those who want to build 'real world' strength and conditioning
- Those without the time to attend the gym
- Those without access to a gym
- Athletes - especially those involved in contact sports e.g. MMA, Judo, Rugby, American Football
- Those who dislike the commercial gym environment
- Those who want to incorporate the benefits of sandbag training into their existing exercise programme

I train at home, in my garage, with minimal equipment. This training guide is designed to support others who want to do this, and also for those who just want to get the benefits of training with sandbags.

Connect With Us

Watch videos, follow the daily workouts and post your times on the Sandbag Fitness blog.
www.sandbagfitness.blogspot.com

We post all of our workouts on our Facebook page.
www.facebook.com/sandbagfitness

We're always looking to connect with people following the workouts so if you've got pictures of your garage gym or video of you training then we'd love to see them too.
matthewpalfrey@gmail.com

My Youtube channel has some useful instructional video for Sandbag Fitness.
www.youtube.com/user/CoachPalfrey

The Sandbag Fitness Store has a range of sandbag training products and services.
www.sandbagfitnessstore.com

The Benefits of Sandbag Training

This thing is awkward to lift

For me, the greatest benefit of the sandbag is the fact that it is awkward to lift. The load is constantly shifting, or at least requires effort to stabilise, and this produces an effect far removed from conventional weight training. The sandbag is not ergonomically designed to make it easier to lift – it makes you work hard for each repetition. The result is that you build strength and conditioning that can be applied in the real world. Scientists would call this 'ecological validity'.

This concept of functional strength is heavily touted in modern health and fitness. It's not uncommon to find classic exercises 'modified' to include instability by using stability balls, boards and another equipment. But the sandbag has built-in instability, making it the natural choice to integrate instability training into your programme.

The major advantage of training with an unstable object, rather than on an unstable surface, is that it has greater ecological validity or real world application. Most loads, in real life, are not equally weighted. Therefore, training with the sandbag prepares the body to deal with an unstable load. The 'craze' for stability training typically involves making the surface on which you are standing unstable – the complete opposite of most real world situations.

The Benefits of Sandbag Training

Have bag, will travel

If you travel regularly, as I do, then the sandbag is a great addition to any suitcase. I take mine with me everywhere I go and fill it when I arrive – either at the beach or from a builder's merchant. It is the ultimate portable gym so you have no excuses not to train again!

Value For Money

The sandbag is proudly low-tech and relatively inexpensive compared to other training options. In a comparison of cost between sand and conventional weight plates the sand comes in at around 1/20th of the price. And that's if you pay for it – sand is fairly easy to come by for free. I have around 200kgs/440lbs of sand in my garage gym and this cost me about £15/$24 – the same weight in even the most basic plates would have set me back at least £300/$450, and that's without the bars and collars.

With so many barriers to exercise, the inexpensive nature of sandbag training makes it a great option for everyone.

The Benefits of Sandbag Training

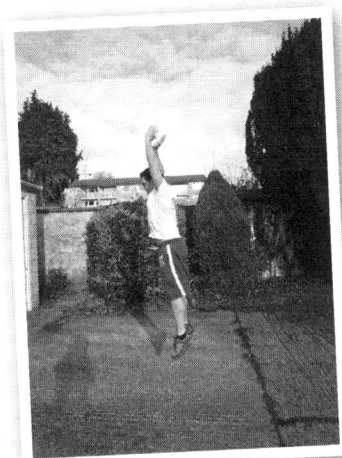

Bend me, shape me

The sandbag is malleable – it will mould itself to your body and most shapes you can think of. I've seen countless attempts to make barbell back squats more comfortable with towels, various ergonomic pads and even extra t-shirts but the sandbag will mould itself nicely across your upper back – problem solved.

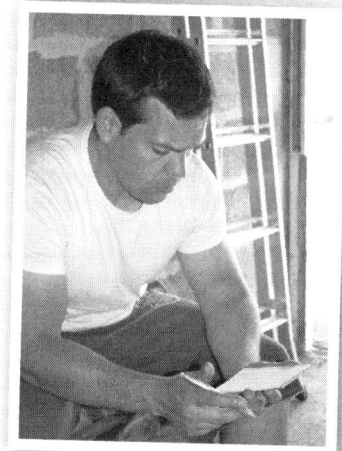

The malleable sandbag also lends itself well to load carries, hill sprints and various sport specific drills. I find it particularly effective with combat athletes as the bag can be used to simulate an opponent effectively.

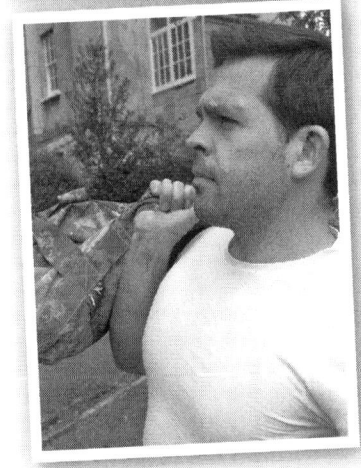

The sandbag can take the place of a medicine ball for throwing, passing and catching drills – try doing that with a barbell.

The Benefits of Sandbag Training

Get a grip

Most modern gymnasiums are littered with machines that require little to no hand strength to operate them. This causes problems when, outside of the gym, you require hand strength to lift anything. The modern antidote to this problem is to include some additional grip strength exercises to supplement your grip-independent strength workout. The sandbag avoids this unnecessary issue by requiring high levels of grip strength to lift – it builds hand and forearm conditioning naturally.

Grip strength is a vital attribute for all athletes – especially Wrestlers, MMA fighters and contact sportspeople. It's also important for the population as a whole. You only have to consider the commercial market for grip assistance implements to see how much of a problem this is becoming in modern society. Regular practice with a sandbag would maintain grip strength into old age.

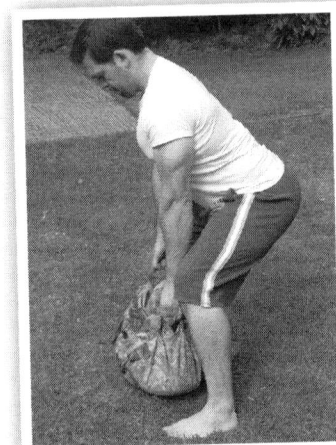

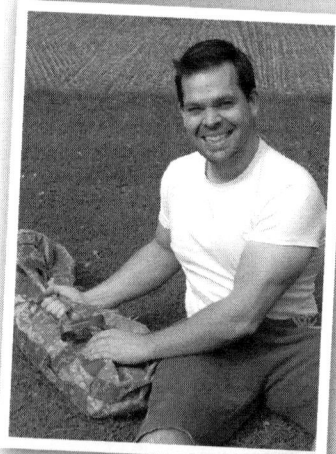

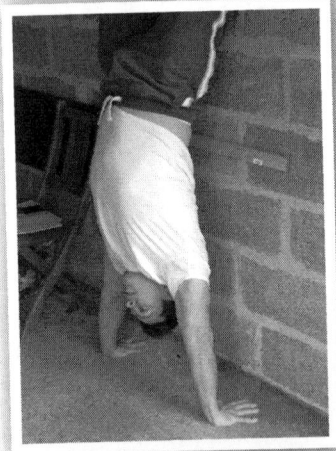

Equipment

I developed Sandbag Fitness and the Complete Guide To Sandbag Training as a cost-effective alternative to traditional gym membership or exercise class - I really wanted to show that it's possible to achieve great results with the minimum of investment.

When I started out it was just me, a 25kg/55lb sandbag and a pull up bar. As time has gone on I've added a few other things that have really helped with my overall progress. If you do want to invest in some additional equipment then I'll recommend the best available options.

Sandbags

These will generally fall into one of two categories - homemade or custom-made. Homemade bags are cheaper than custom-made bags but nowhere near as versatile.

Over the page you'll find the pro's and con's for both options.

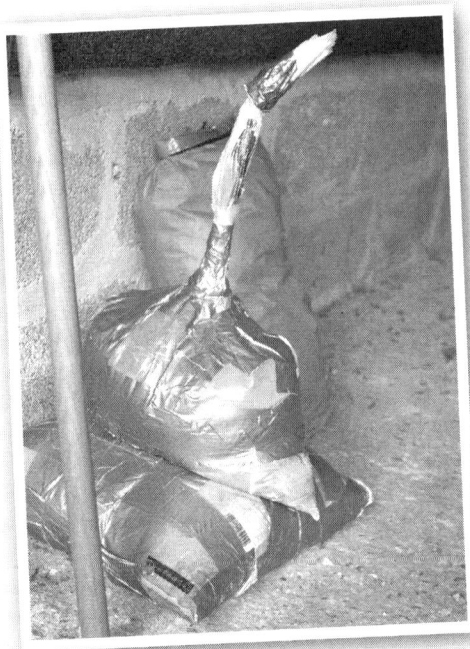

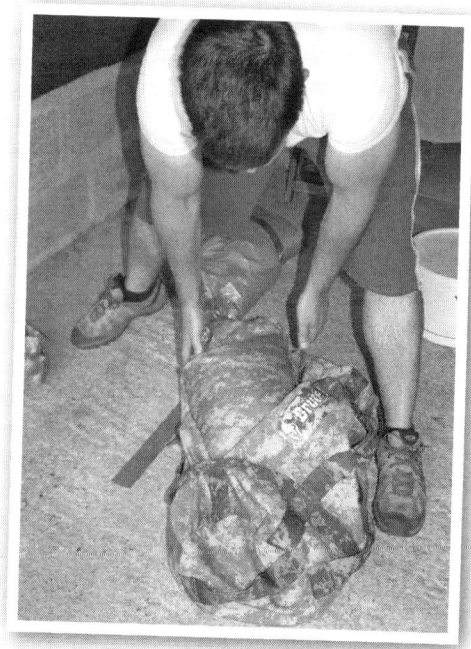

Equipment

Homemade Sandbags

The quickest and cheapest way to get started is with a bag of sand from a hardware store or builders merchant - this is how I started. Get the size/weight that you want or split a bag if you need to. Liberally apply some tape and you're ready to go. You should also put this sandbag into a larger, more robust 'outer' bag. This can stop the sandbag splitting when you are lifting it. I have used waterproof 'stuff-sacks' and holdalls for this purpose and they work pretty well.

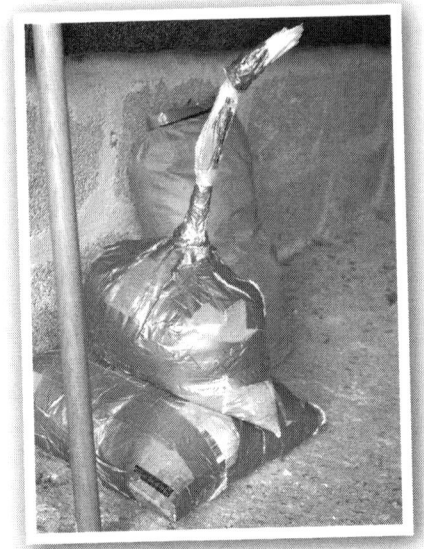

My original range of bags contained the following:

1. A homemade 'tornado ball' made from a half sack of sand (about 9kg/20lb) and lots of tape.

2. A 25kg/55lb bag of sand inside a waterproof 'stuff-sack'.

3. An old rucksack filled with 2-3 25kg bags of sand.

While you can complete the workouts with just one bag it is more convenient to have a light, medium and heavy bag and the 'tornado ball' is also good to have on hand.

People can get quite hung up on how to make their sandbag but I've found it's generally best to leave the sand in its original bag and put it into another bag of some kind.

Equipment

Custom-made Sandbags

The custom-made sandbag will normally have three major advantages over the homemade bag:

1. It has handles, making movements like Rows, Pulls and Deadlifts much more effective.

2. It will be more hardwearing than the homemade sandbag.

3. It will have 'filler' bags, making it easy to adjust the weight from exercise to exercise or session to session. These can also be used as sandbags in their own right (please note that they are not designed for this).

I only train with the Brute Force Sandbag. Their products and service are second to none.

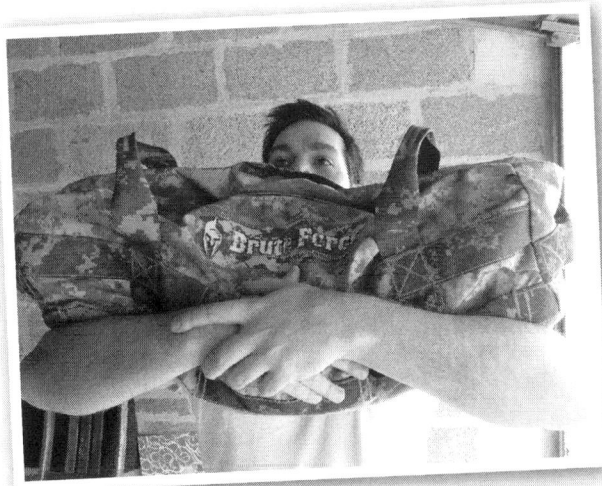

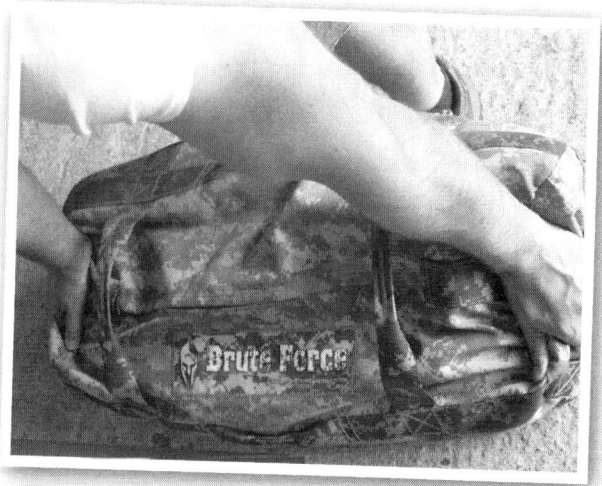

Equipment

Pull Up Bar

You're going to need something that you can hang from, ideally at arms length, to perform Pull Ups, Knees-to Elbows, Hanging Leg Raises and Toes-to-Bar. This could be a tree branch, climbing frame, ledge or something homemade. My pull up bar consists of a bar attached to the beams of my garage via 2 hooks.

You can also use Gymnastic Rings - with the added benefit that you can adjust the height to perform supine rows (australian pull ups) if you need to. The guys at Ring Training, make the best rings available.

Another alternative is the TRX - this portable suspension trainer is highly recommended.

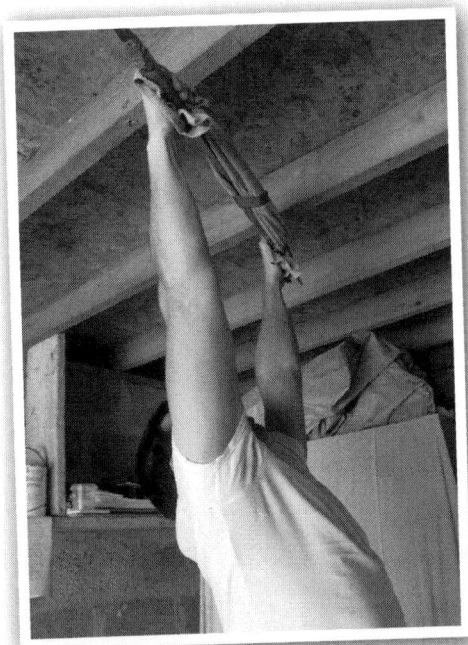

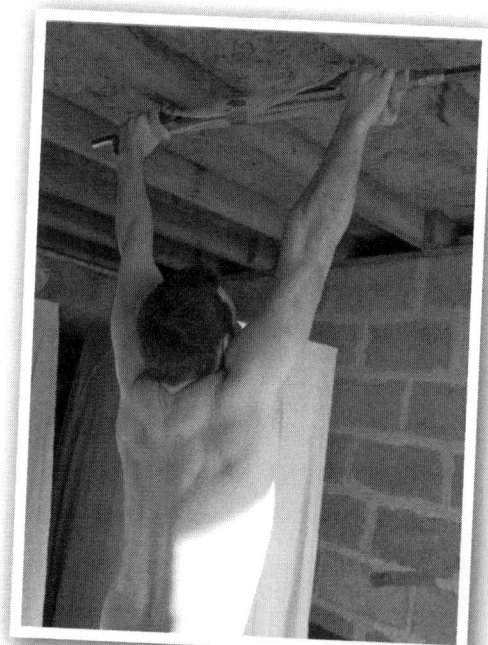

Equipment

Box/Platform

I constructed a platform for box jumps from a box and a couple of sandbags. You can use any sturdy platform - ideally around 20 - 30 inches high.

Timing

You'll also needs some method of timing your workouts. If you don't already have something suitable the Gymboss timer is an excellent option - and perfect for interval training.

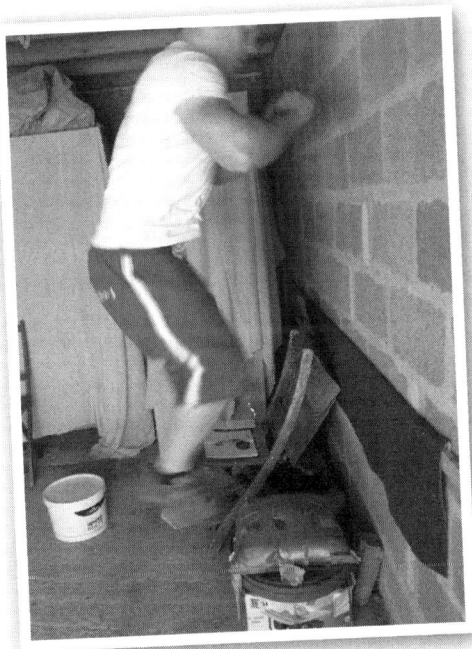

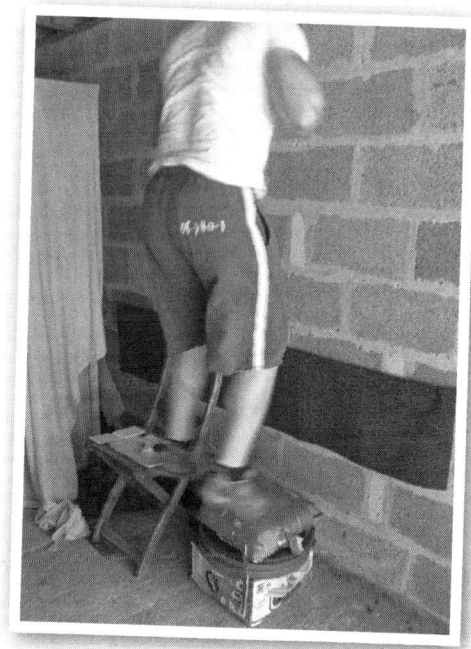

Equipment Checklist

Sandbag

- Use a homemade sandbag made from a holdall or duffel bag
- Get a custom made sandbag from Brute Force Sandbags

Pull Up Bar

- Use any sturdy bar, climbing frame or tree branch
- Get some Gymnastic Rings
- Get a TRX

Box/Platform

- Use any sturdy platform around 20-30" high

Timer

- Use a stopwatch
- Get a Gymboss Timer

You can purchase all of this equipment through the Sandbag Fitness blog 'Store' page

http://sandbagfitness.blogspot.co.uk/p/store.html

Making This Programme Work

The basis behind sound, progressive exercise is actually pretty simple. Unfortunately, it's easy to get caught up in the huge number of options available to todays modern trainee. We are bombarded with so many options that it can be overwhelming. My advice is that you should view everything you do not as an arbitrary goal but with the mindset of getting good at exercise. Practice the exercises and you'll get better.

Apply Performance Indicators - And Stick To Them

One of the major reasons that people fail to stick to their training programme is that they don't chart performance changes. But this failure happens at the very start.

If you are following this, or any other programme, with the belief that you will achieve miracles then you should re-think things. You can get great results from the programmes and exercises contained in this guide - but it takes hard work and dedication.

For each and every session you do, record your performance. Get yourself a notebook or print the programme section and leave it next to your sandbag - that way you'll be reminded each time you train.

Making This Programme Work

What you record will depend on the workout for that day but it will generally include:

- The time taken to complete a set workload
- Your "score" for a given challenge
- The weight of the sandbag you used for the workout
- Rest periods, if applicable

It could also include the following:

- The "level" of the exercise - did you do it as recommended or was it adapted to make it harder or easier
- The quality of each exercise - use this as a guide for future technique
- How tough the session was
- Variations of the exercise - grip used, position of the sandbag

This record book of your performance is vital to allow you to keep progressing, give you targets for each session and help you to avoid plateaus.

The number of people I speak to who do not record what they do each time they train is staggering. Recording the details of each session is also important as a means to measure "actual" progress versus "implied" progress. It's easy to make 'progress' if the goalposts are constantly being moved:

- Are you maintaining the quality of each exercise?
- For a given workload, are you taking longer rest periods?

How To Grip
The Sandbag

Resistance training in general is good for grip strength. The sandbag can be a particularly effective grip training tool because it is a challenge to hold on to. People often ask me how they should be holding the sandbag - and the honest answer is that there is no right or wrong way. In order to challenge your grip I recommend utilising a variety of different grips, either between exercises or from session to session. And it is important to remember that gripping needn't involve using your hands - any contact with the bag can be classed as a grip.

What you'll find is that the sandbag can be much more versatile than the average free weight.

Below you'll find some of the most common grips that I use.

Common Grips

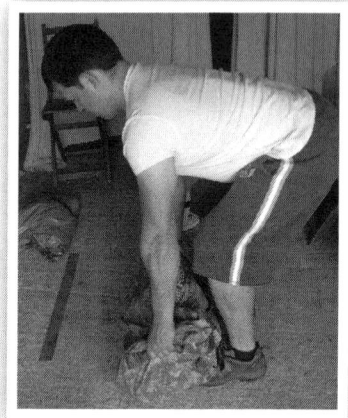

Bag Grip

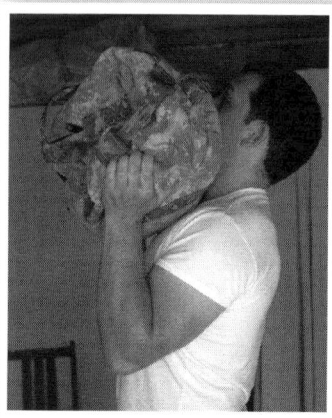

Bag Grip

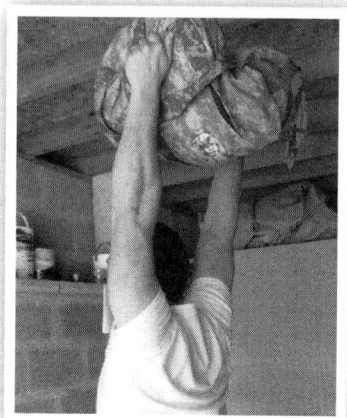

Bag Grip

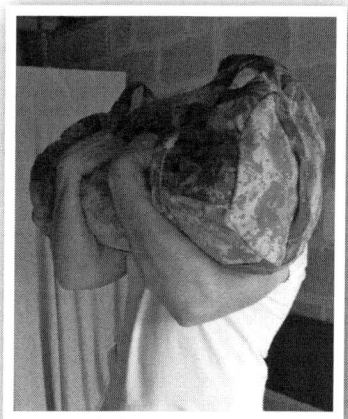

Zercher Grip

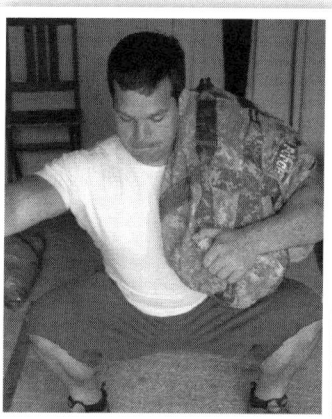

Shoulder Grip

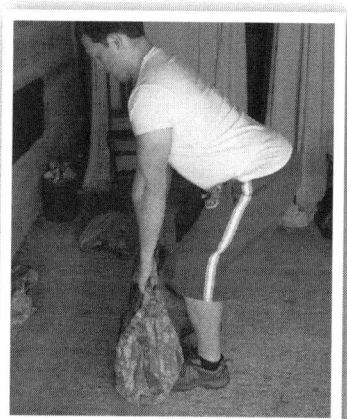

Horizontal Handles

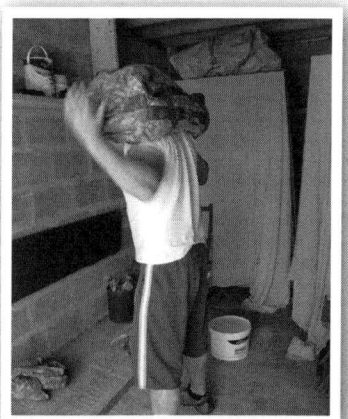

Across the Shoulders

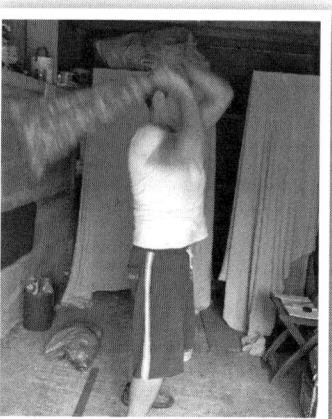

Filler Grip

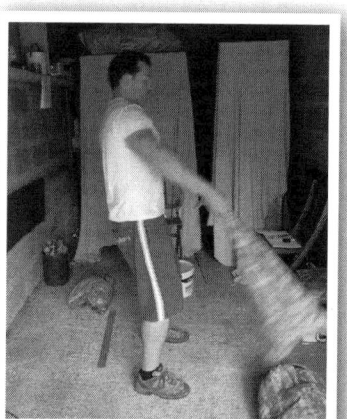

Single arm Filler Grip

Warm Ups

Prior to starting any exercise I suggest you take some time to warm up and prepare yourself physically and mentally for the workout ahead. A good warm up will help to improve performance, reduce the chance of injury and improve recovery time.

At Sandbag Fitness we follow a simple approach to warming up - lots of movement, a few stretches and some light practice of the movements that are going to be in the workout for that day.

Warm Ups

Warm Up Routine

1. 2-4 minutes light skipping or a jog.

2. 20 Shoulder Rolls.

Take a broomstick or PVC pipe and hold with a wide grip. Keeping your arms straight, raise the bar upwards and above your head. If possible move the bar all the way down towards your lower back. This is best achieved with a shoulder shrug at the top of the movement. If you can do this easily then take a narrower grip on the bar and repeat.

3. Squat Stretch for 1-2 minutes.

Sit down into a deep squat and, using your elbows, push your knees outwards until you feel a stretch in the groin.

4. Lunge Stretch for 30-60 seconds on each leg.

Holding the broomstick or PVC pipe overhead, take a big lunge step forwards. Hold this position for 30-60 seconds. Repeat on the opposite leg.

5. 2-4 minutes practice of the movements for that days workout.

6. Bar Hang for 30-60 seconds.

7. Workout!

Warm Ups

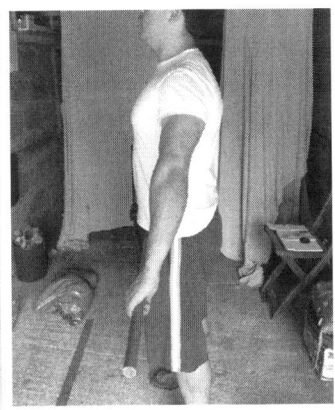

Shoulder Rolls

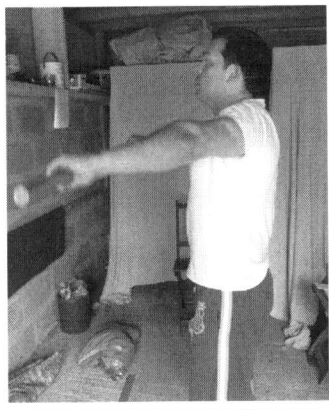

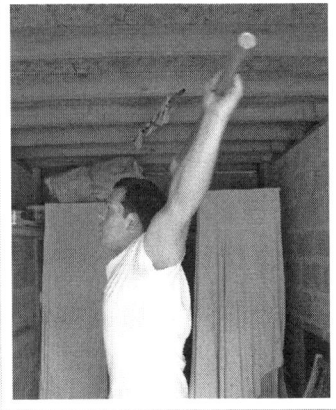

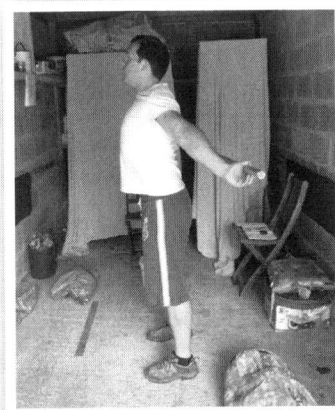

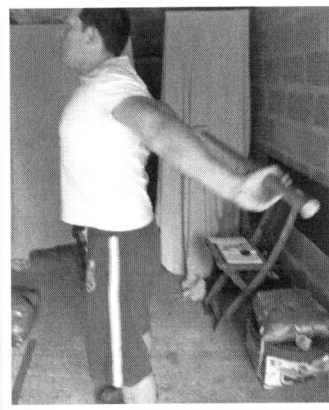

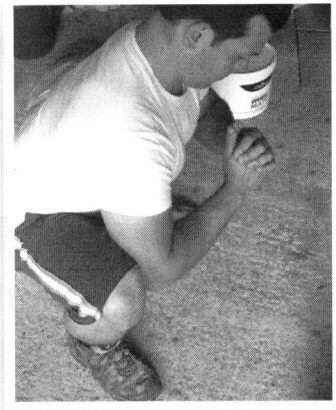

Shoulder Rolls

Shoulder Rolls

Shoulder Rolls

Shoulder Rolls

Squat Stretch

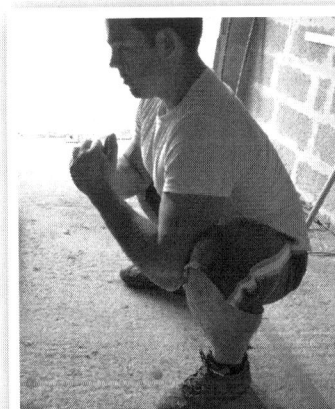

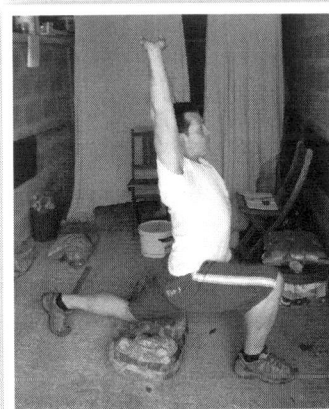

Squat Stretch

Lunge Stretch

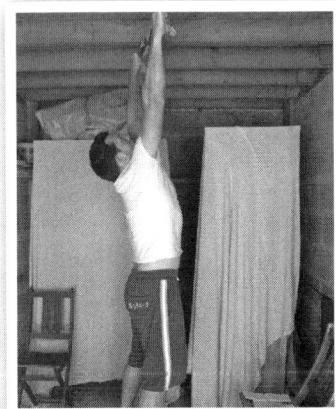

Bar Hang

The Exercises

This guide contains detailed descriptions of the exercises in the Sandbag Fitness training programme. These are the exercises that we use regularly on the Sandbag Fitness Blog. They are also the exercises that you will need to master to be able to complete the programmes contained in this training guide.

At Sandbag Fitness we generally focus on compound movements - big exercises that utilise multiple muscles and joints for "more bang for your buck". I have found that basing the programme around these movements produces the best results in the least time. The programme also contains both sandbag exercises and bodyweight exercises. Why? Because it is important to develop the ability to master your own bodyweight too.

The exercises are divided into sections by movement pattern:

- **Squat and Lunge**
- **Deadlift**
- **Press**
- **Pull**
- **Core**
- **Full Body**

This will make it easier for you to construct your own programme if you require. Please note: while the exercises have been categorized this way, many of the exercises work multiple muscle groups.

If there are some terms that you are not familiar with be sure to check the Glossary.

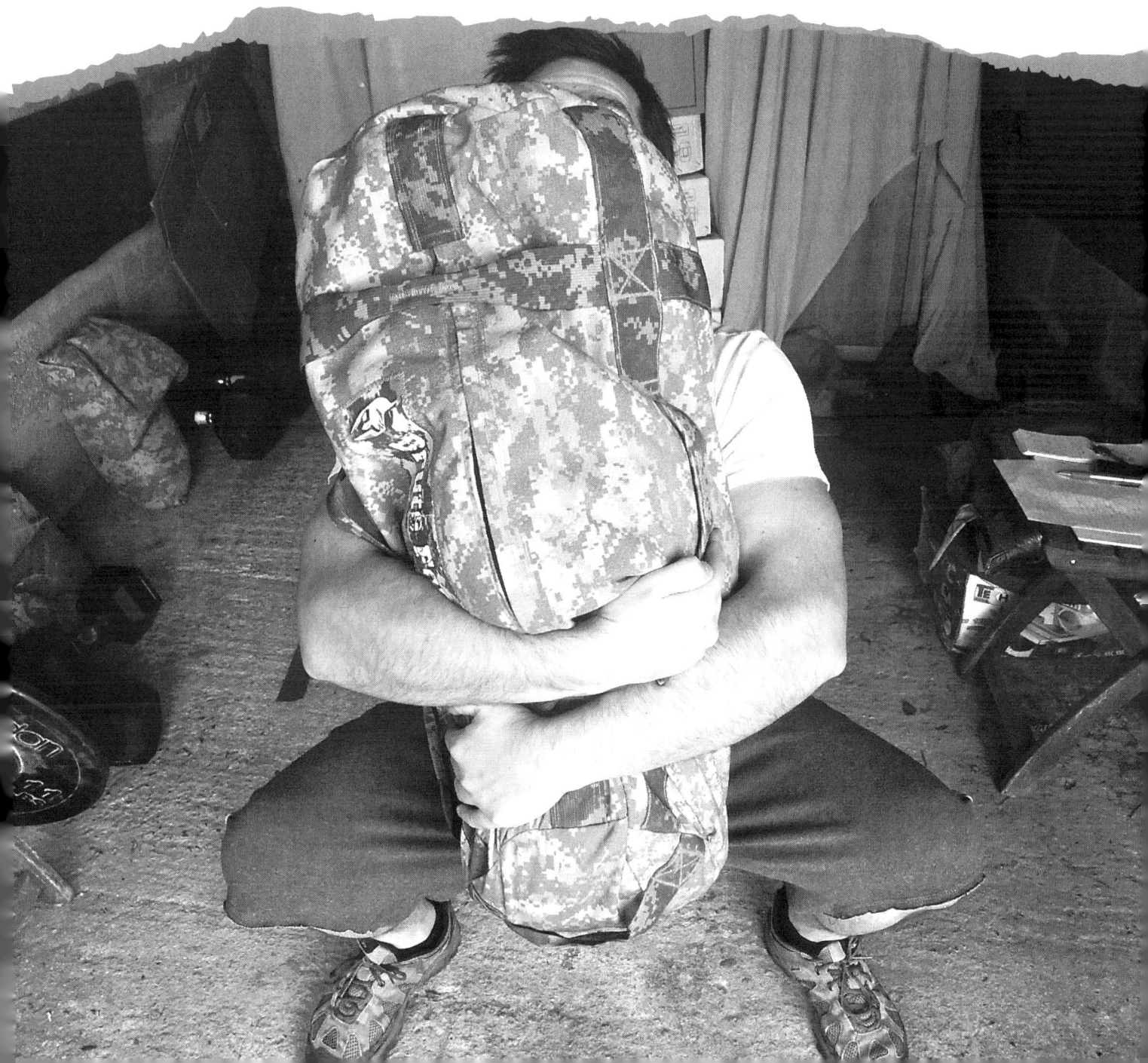

SQUAT
& LUNGE

Sandbag Back Squat

The Sandbag Back Squat is one of our top 3 strength building exercises, the others being the Sandbag Deadlift and the Sandbag Overhead Press. At Sandbag Fitness we perform it exactly (with just a few small adjustments) as you would with a regular Barbell. The major variations are based around working specifically with the bag as opposed to the bar. With that in mind, you could use the sandbag back squat as part of a modified Starting Strength or Wendler 5-3-1 programme.

The Sandbag Back Squat is the squat variation that will allow you to lift the most weight - it is therefore a vital component for building strength. However, we also include Sandbag Front Squats, Sandbag Zercher Squats, Sandbag Shoulder Squats and Sandbag Bear Hug Squats in this programme for the other benefits they provide.

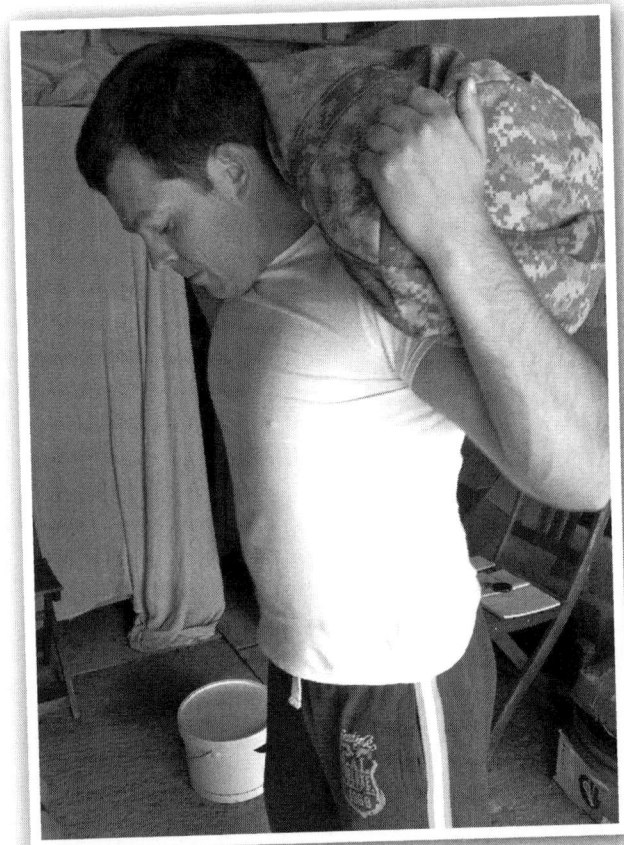

Sandbag Back Squat

Technique

- The first challenge is to get the sandbag up onto your back - I normally Clean and Press it into position
- The sandbag should sit horizontally across your upper back - use your hands and traps to keep it in place
- Your feet should be at least shoulder width apart and slightly turned out
- Begin the movement by pushing your hips back into the squat
- Bend your knees and squat down so your knees are at least parallel with the crease in your hip
- Drive the hips back upwards and return to standing
- The chest should stay fairly high
- Feet should stay flat with the weight predominantly in the rear of the foot
- The knees can track forward but try to avoid them passing excessively in front of the toes
- The knees should remain in-line with the feet at all times - do not allow the knees to track inwards toward each other

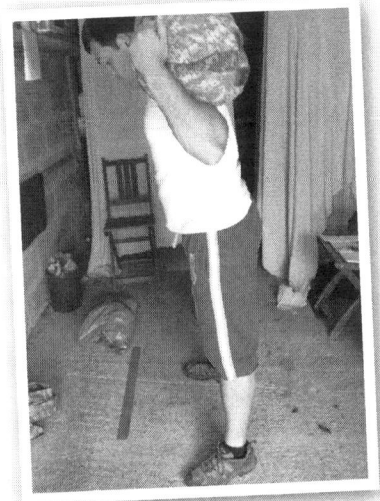

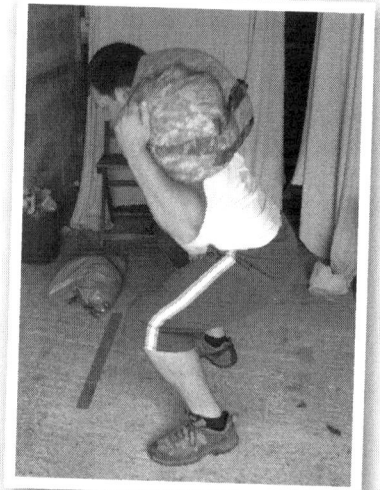

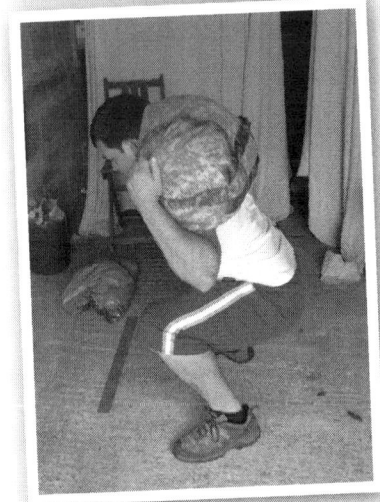

Sandbag Front Squat

The Sandbag Front Squat is a variation that won't allow you to lift as much weight as the more common Sandbag Back Squat. It is, however, a vital functional movement and requires a higher degree of core strength than other squat variations. I say functional because it is a more natural (and likely) position in which be holding an external weight. It also progresses nicely into Press variations and the Sandbag Clean.

Technique

- Get the sandbag up to chest height - either Clean it or "anyhow" lift
- Keep the elbows under the sandbag
- Sit back into the squat as normal
- Try to remain more upright than in a back squat
- Try to stay in neutral spine throughout the movement
- Drive the hips back upwards and return to standing
- The chest should stay fairly high
- Feet should stay flat with the weight predominantly in the rear of the foot
- The knees can track forward but try to avoid them passing excessively in front of the toes
- The knees should remain in-line with the feet at all times - do not allow the knees to track inwards toward each other

Sandbag Front Squat

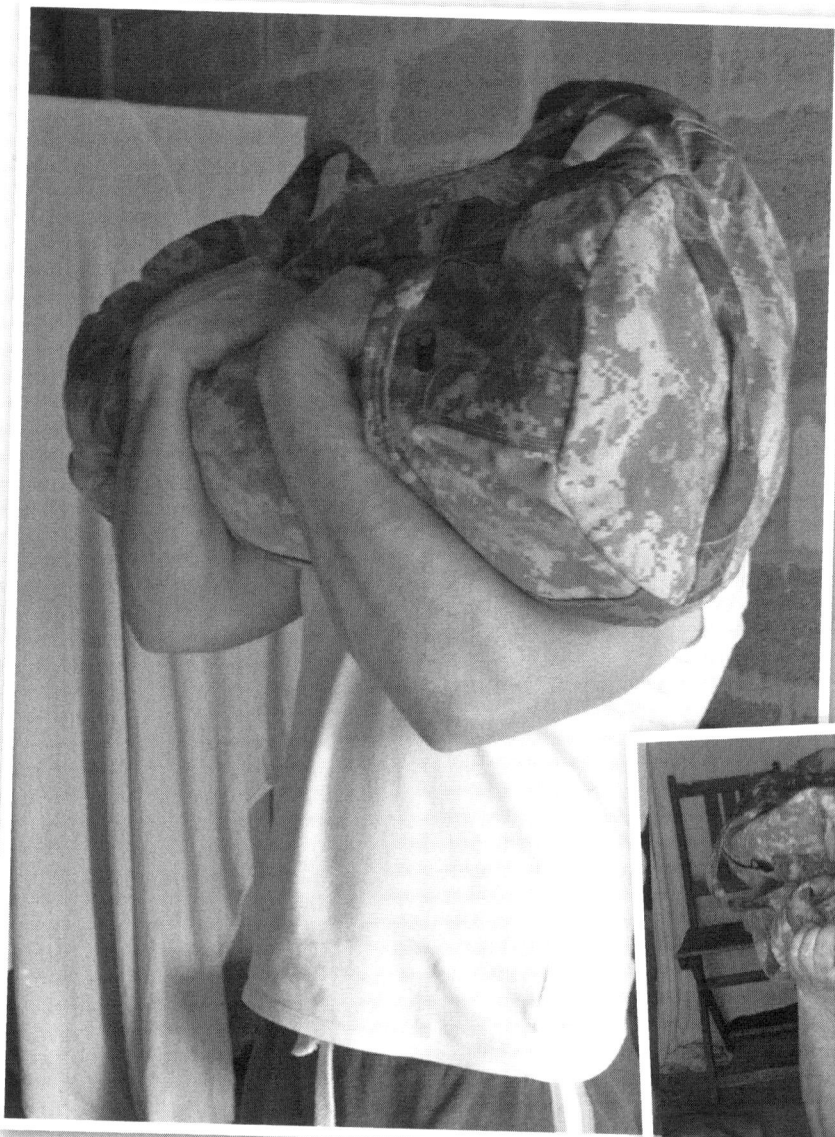

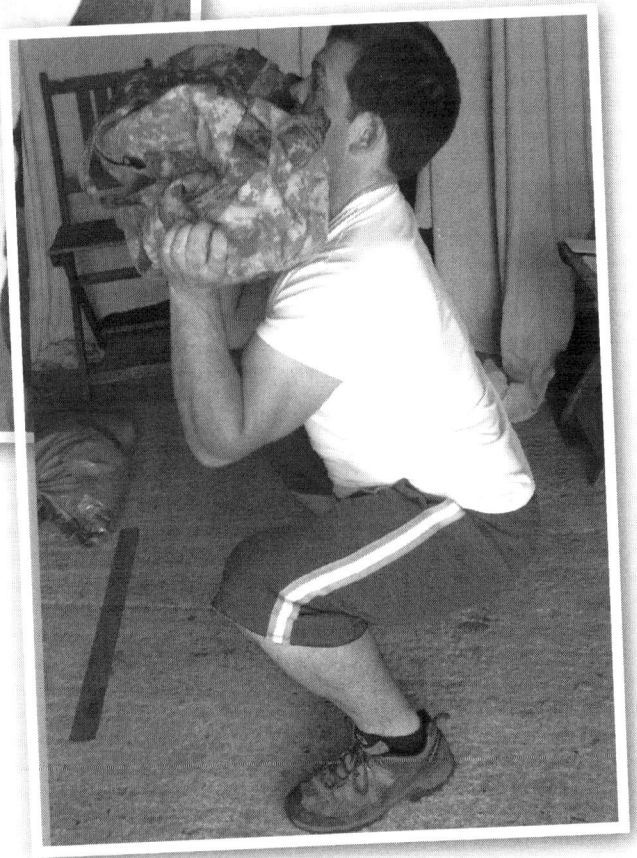

Sandbag Zercher Squat

The Sandbag Zercher Squat is a front squat variation and refers to the grip used. The sandbag is held in the 'crook' of the arms. It is a tough exercise that requires great upper body and core strength.

Technique

- Get the sandbag up to chest height - either Clean it or "anyhow" lift
- Sit back into the squat as normal
- Try to remain more upright than in a back squat
- Try to stay in neutral spine throughout the movement
- Drive the hips back upwards and return to standing
- The chest should stay fairly high
- Feet should stay flat with the weight predominantly in the rear of the foot
- The knees can track forward but try to avoid them passing excessively in front of the toes
- The knees should remain in-line with the feet at all times - do not allow the knees to track inwards toward each other

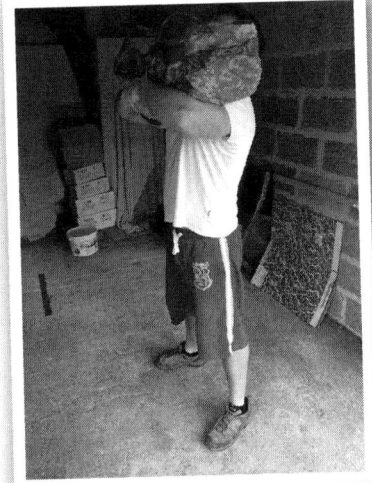

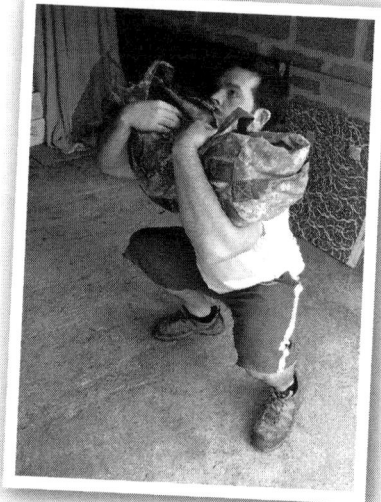

Sandbag Bear Hug Squat

The Sandbag Bear Hug Squat is another front squat variation that places particular demands on core and upper body strength. A highly functional movement for athletes in contact sports, it's also useful for anyone wishing to build strength.

Technique

- Squat down and take a firm bear hug grip around your sandbag
- Sit back into the squat as normal
- Try to remain more upright than in a back squat
- Try to stay in neutral spine throughout the movement
- Drive the hips back upwards and return to standing
- Feet should stay flat with the weight predominantly in the rear of the foot
- The knees can track forward but try to avoid them passing excessively in front of the toes
- The knees should remain in-line with the feet at all times - do not allow the knees to track inwards toward each other

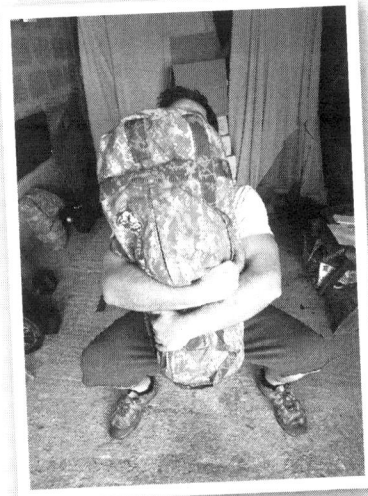

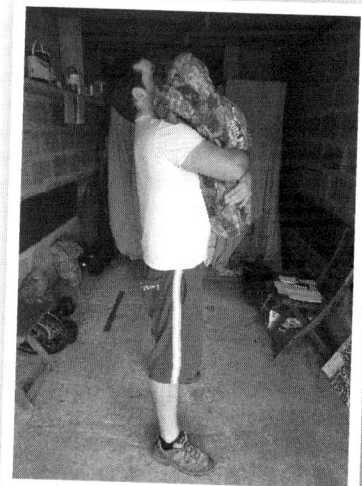

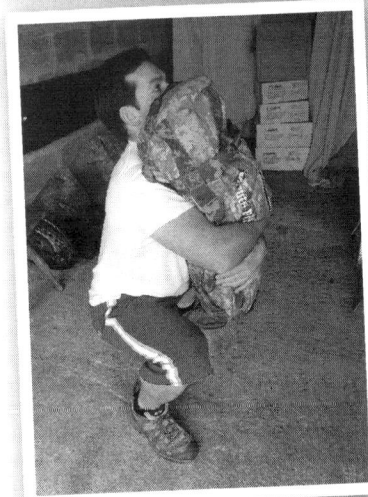

Sandbag Shoulder Squat

The Sandbag Shoulder Squat places additional demands on the core and your lateral stability.

Technique

- Lift the sandbag up onto your shoulder
- Sit back into the squat as normal
- Try to remain more upright than in a back squat
- Try to stay in neutral spine throughout the movement
- Drive the hips back upwards and return to standing
- Feet should stay flat with the weight predominantly in the rear of the foot
- The knees can track forward but try to avoid them passing excessively in front of the toes
- The knees should remain in-line with the feet at all times - do not allow the knees to track inwards toward each other

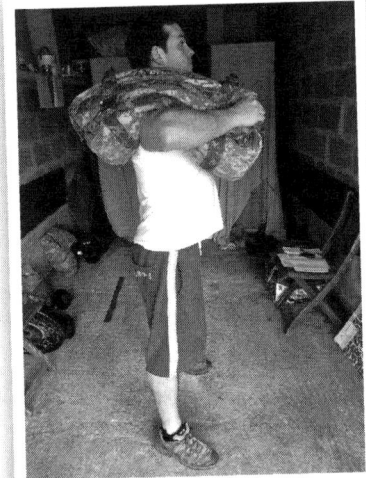

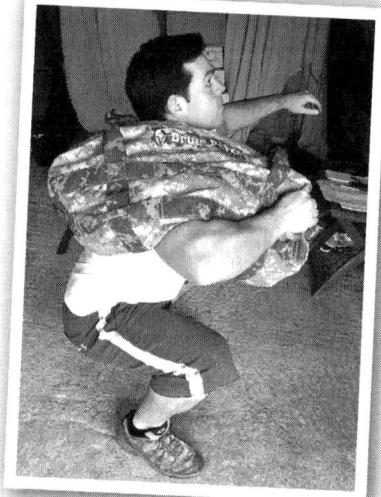

Sandbag Lunge

The Sandbag Lunge is a good exercise for building strength in the lower body. It's also a versatile exercise with a number of variations.

Technique

- Lift the sandbag up onto your shoulders
- Step forward on one leg
- Bend both knees and drop your bodyweight downwards until both knees are at 90°
- Keep the head and chest high throughout
- Return to the start position and repeat on the opposite side

Variations

- Hold the sandbag in a Zercher or Overhead position
- Perform a Sandbag Walking Lunge by stepping forwards after each lunge

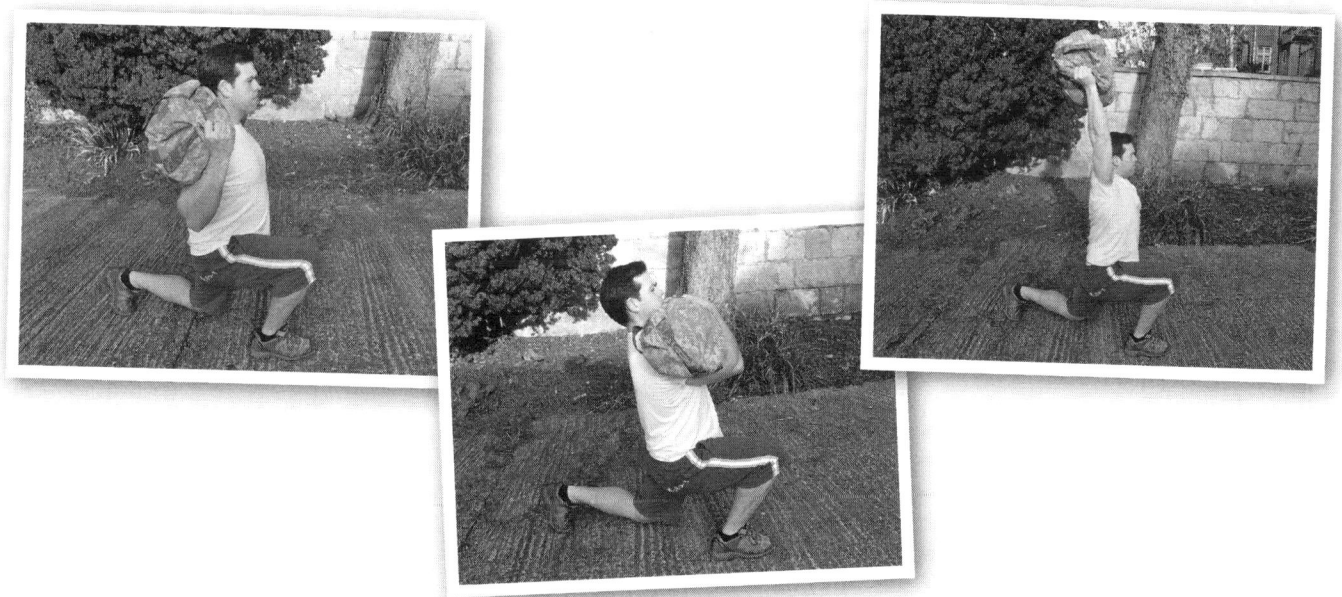

Bodyweight or "Air" Squat

This is the basic squat variation and will develop the strength, skill and conditioning you need to progress onto any weighted versions. It is irreplaceable in any exercise programme.

Technique

- Begin by setting your feet in the right position - this is normally about shoulder width apart, with the feet slightly turned out
- The head stays up high
- To initiate the movement, push your hips back and down as though you are sitting down on a chair behind you
- The arms can be used as a counter balance and to keep the chest high
- Keep the weight predominantly in the heels throughout the movement
- Ensure that the knees track in the same direction as the feet
- Stay active through your abdomen and maintain a neutral spine
- Squat all the way down until your hips are below your knees
- Return to the start position, keeping the chest and head high
- Make sure you stand up tall at the end of the squat and extend fully through the hip

Bodyweight or "Air" Squat

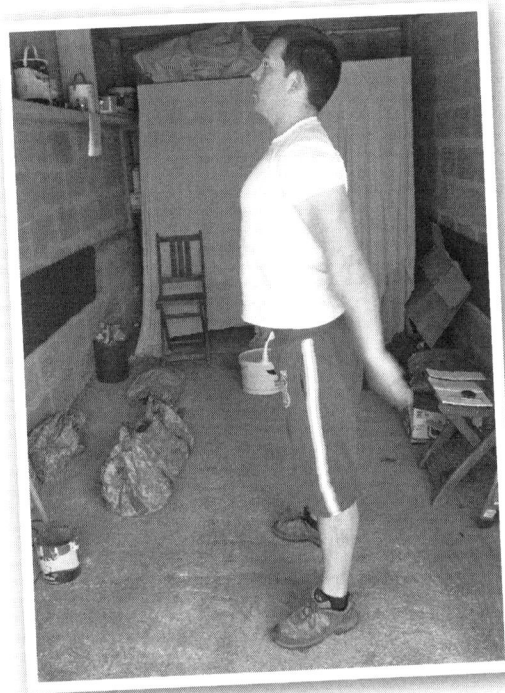

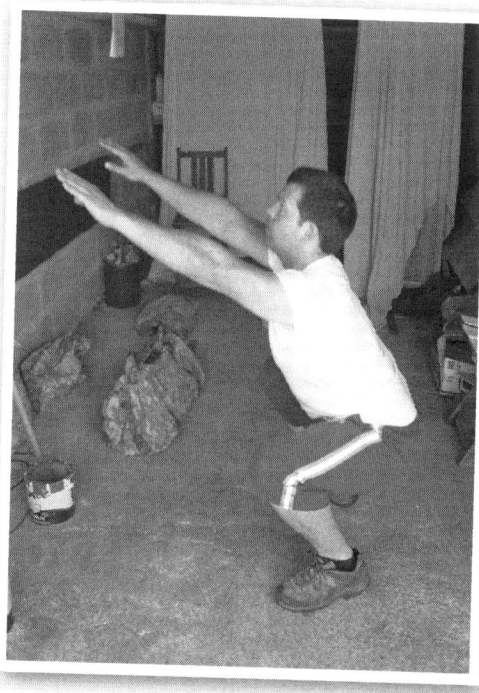

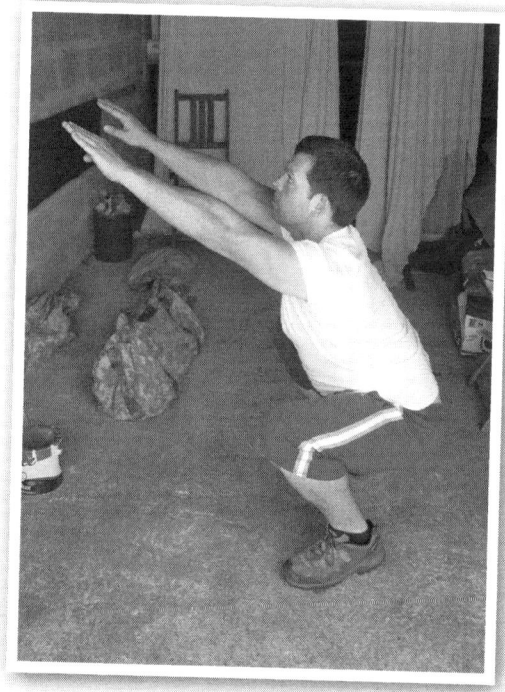

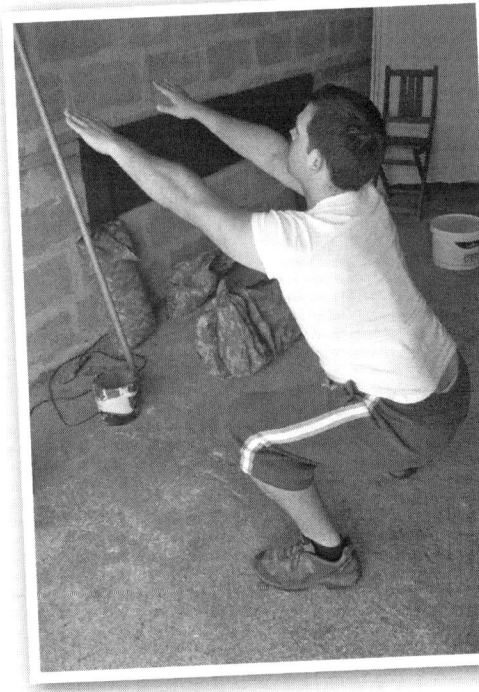

Box Jump

The Box Jump will develop agility and power with a particular focus on the lower body.

Technique

- Stand feet shoulder width apart in front of your box or platform
- Jump explosively upwards, high enough to land on top of the box/platform
- Try to land with flat feet
- Cushion the landing with a slight knee bend
- Explode back upwards and off the box/platform - making sure to get a full hip extension in between each jump
- Cushion the landing back on the floor and repeat
- Use the arms to aid momentum

Variations

- Make the exercise easier by stepping up onto the box rather than jumping - but make sure to complete the required number of repetitions on each leg
- You can also make it easier by using a lower box/platform
- Make the exercise harder with a higher platform or by adding weight

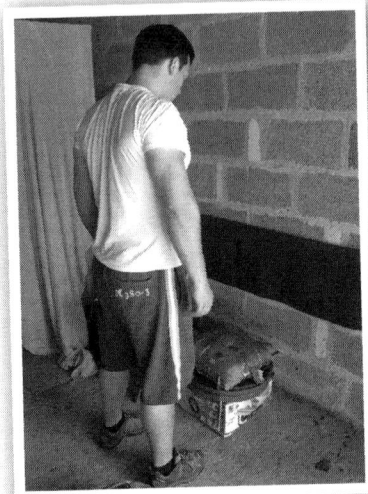

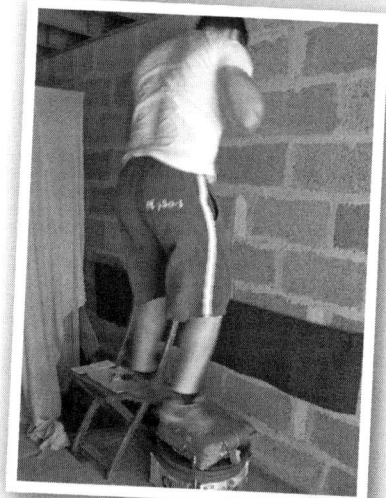

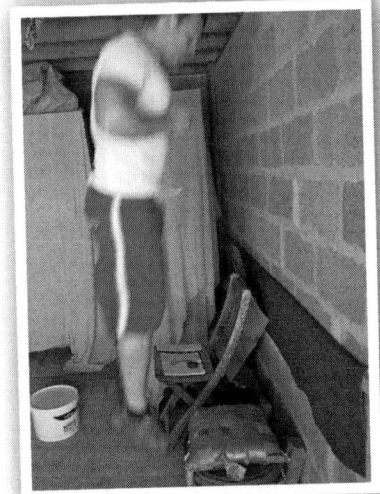

Walking Lunge

The Walking Lunge is a good exercise for building strength in the lower body.

Technique

- Step forward on one leg
- Bend both knees and drop your bodyweight downwards until both knees are at 90°
- Keep the head and chest high throughout
- Bring your rear leg forwards and step through into another lunge
- Try to avoid resting between lunges - keep the movement smooth and continuous
- Don't allow your body to lean forward excessively

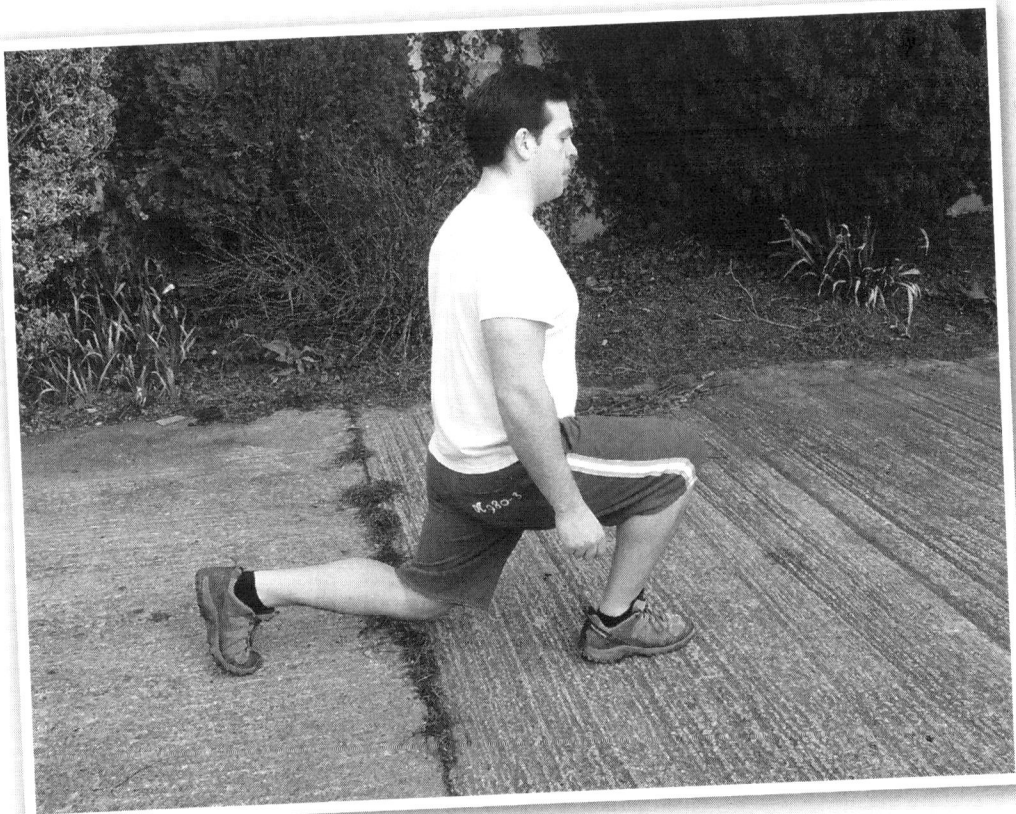

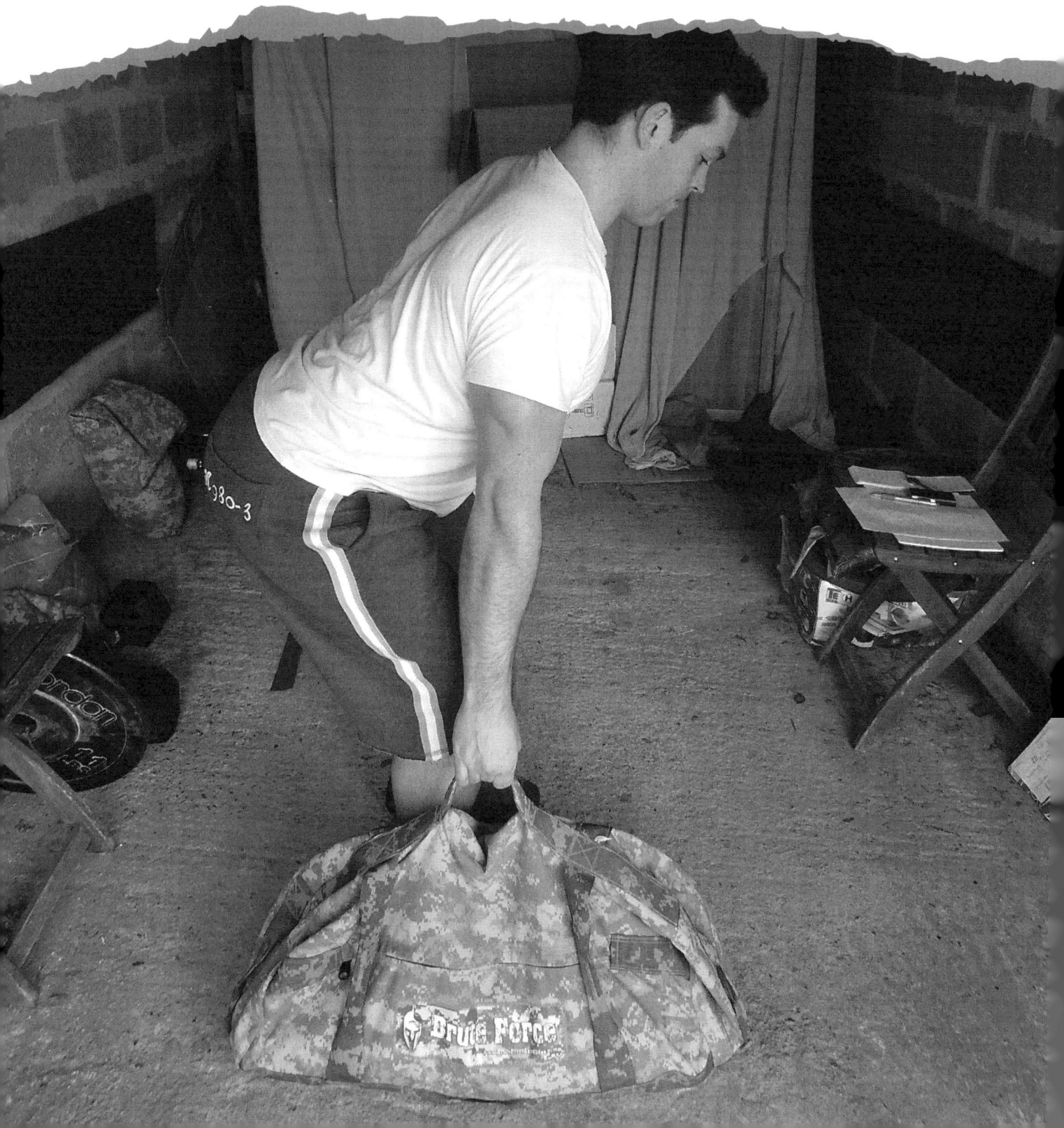

DEADLIFT

Sandbag Deadlift

The Sandbag Deadlift is a key strength movement like the Sandbag Back Squat and the Sandbag Overhead Press. It should be your strongest exercise in terms of the amount of weight you can lift.

Technique

- Start with your feet right next to or under the bag
- Take your grip - this could either be via the handles or the material of the bag
- Set your back in the correct position - neutral spine
- The knees should be slightly bent
- Keep the sandbag close to your legs throughout the lift
- Your shoulders should be over the sandbag
- The arms stay straight - just like hooks
- Maintaining the natural curve in your back, stand upright
- Be sure to open out your hips fully in between lifts

Variations

- See 'Sandbag Suitcase Deadlift'

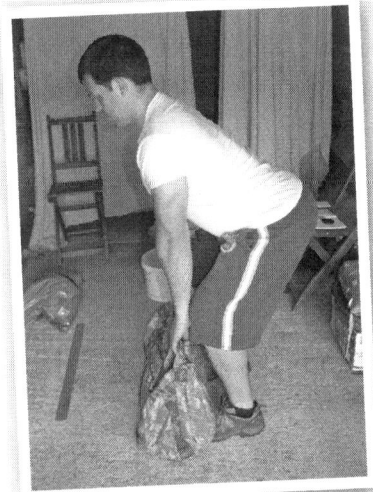

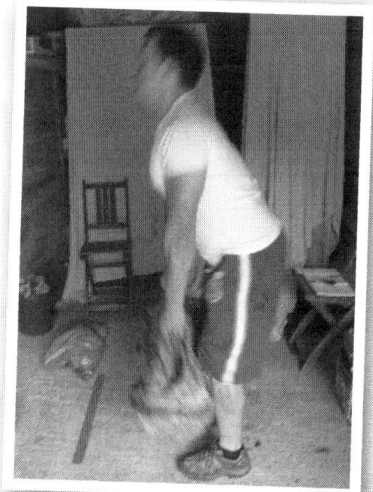

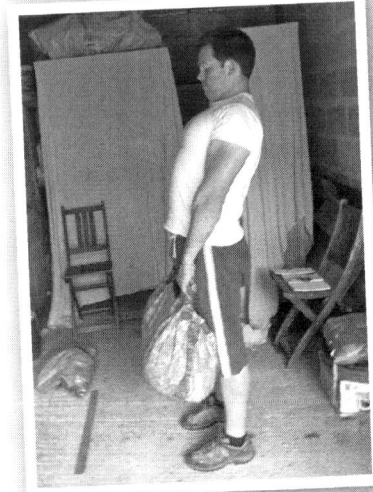

41

Sandbag Suitcase Deadlift

The Suitcase Deadlift is, as the name suggests, similar to lifting a suitcase or bag. The lift is done from the side, placing additional demands on lateral strength and mobility.

Technique

- Start with the sandbag lying horizontal to the side of either foot
- Take your grip - this could either be via the handles or via the material of the bag
- Set your back in the correct position - neutral spine
- The knees should be slightly bent
- Keep the sandbag close to the side of your leg throughout the lift
- The arms stay straight - just like hooks
- Maintaining the natural curve in your back, stand upright
- Be sure to open out your hips fully in between lift

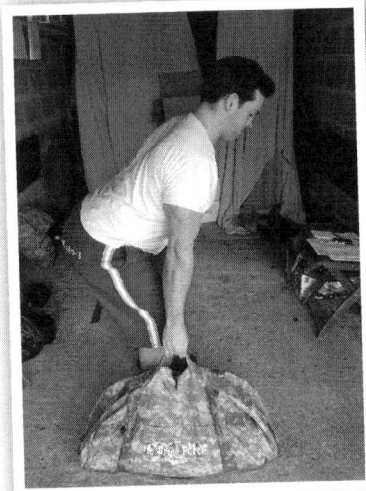

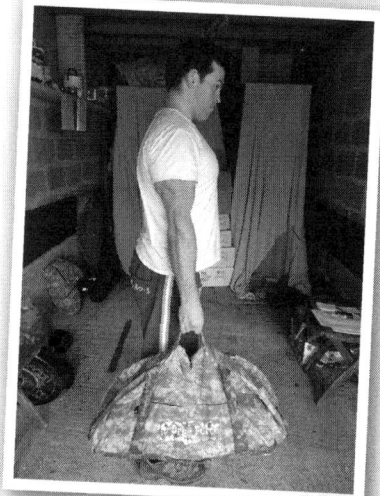

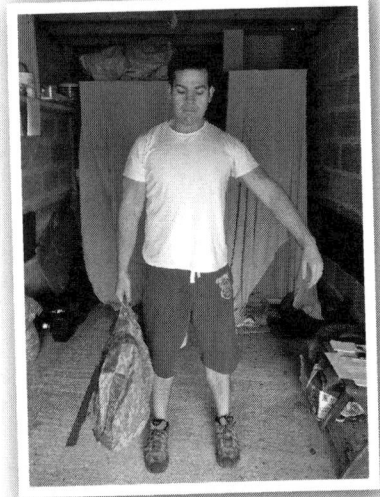

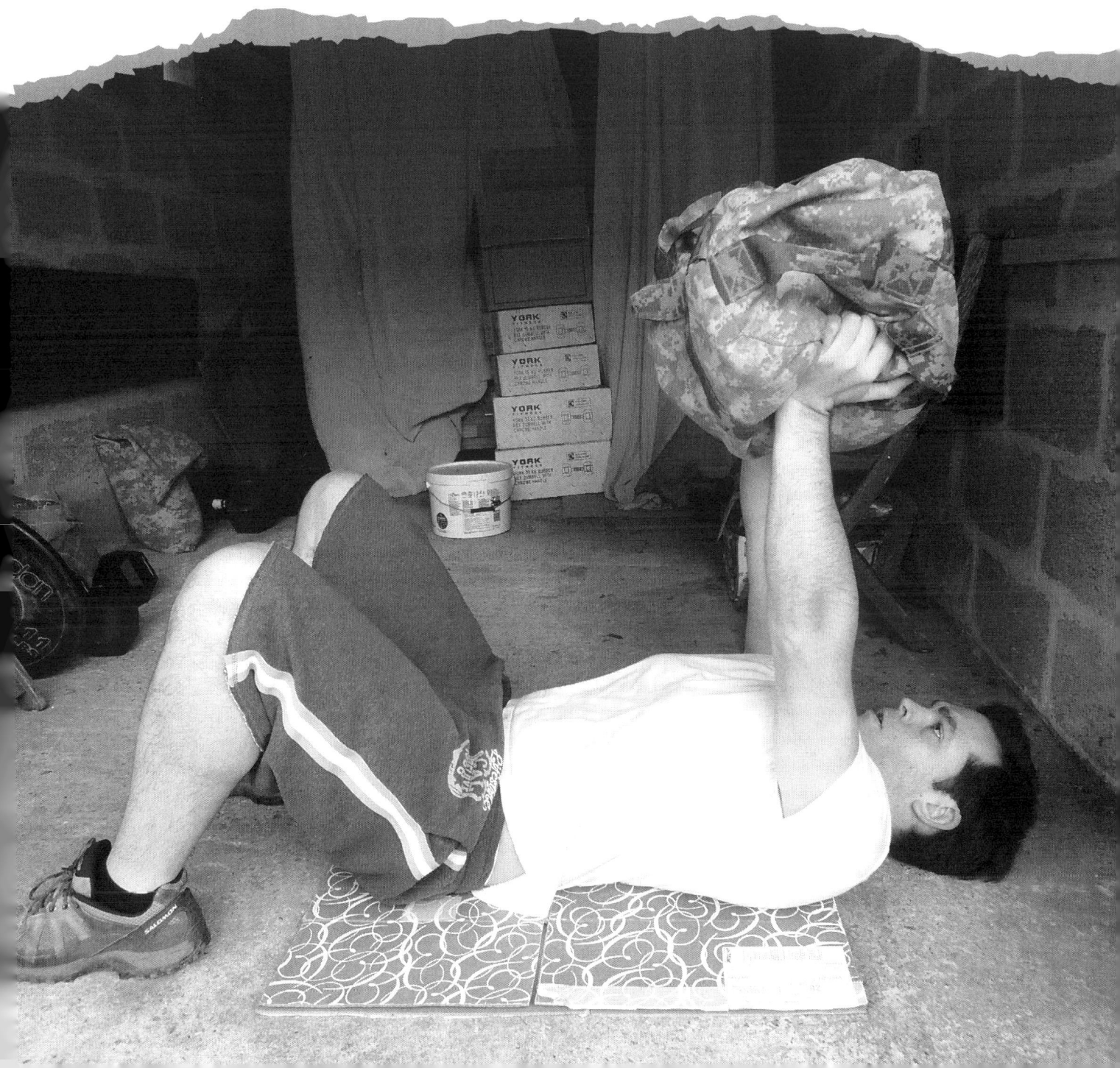

PRESS/
PUSH

Sandbag Overhead Press

The Sandbag Overhead Press is another key movement found in many different programmes like Crossfit, Starting Strength and Wendler 5-3-1. Again, we perform it with few changes - except for the additional challenge of having to stabilise the bag overhead and the different grips needed.

Technique

- Start with the sandbag at chest/shoulder height - as in a front squat
- Without additional help from the legs, press the sandbag upwards and above the head
- The arms should go to full extension
- The head should be slightly in front of the arms at this point of full extension
- Stay in neutral spine throughout
- Return to the starting position and repeat

Variations

- See 'Sandbag Push Press'
- See 'Sandbag Push Jerk'

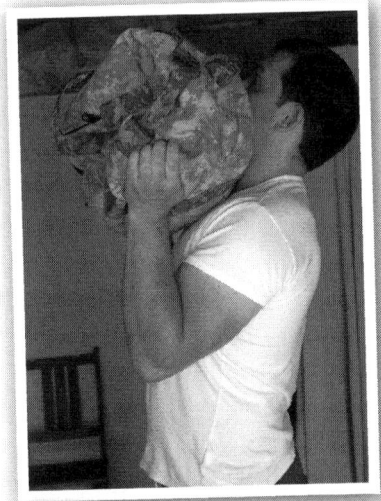

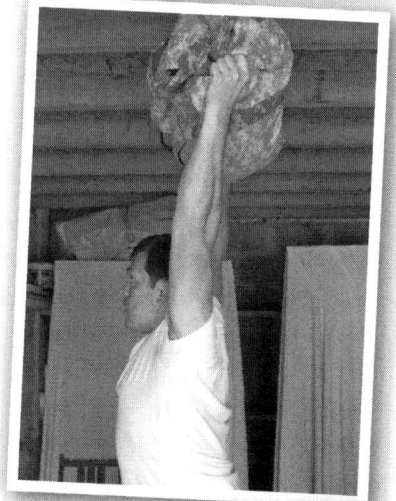

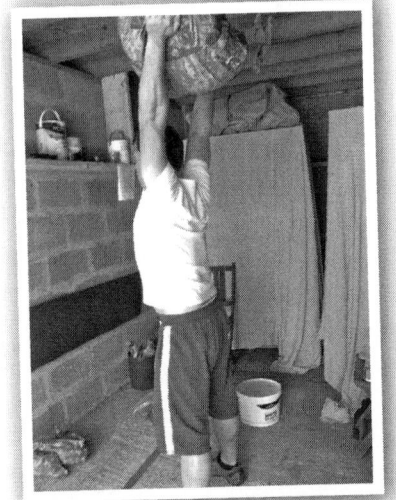

Sandbag Push Press

The Sandbag Push Press is an overhead press variation and a progression onto the Sandbag Push Jerk. Great for developing shoulder power.

Technique

- Start with the sandbag at chest/shoulder height - as in a front squat
- Slightly bend the knees (dip) and then powerfully drive the sandbag overhead - using an extension through both the arms and legs (drive)
- The arms should go to full extension
- The head should be slightly in front of the arms at this point of full extension
- Stay in neutral spine throughout
- Return to the starting position and repeat

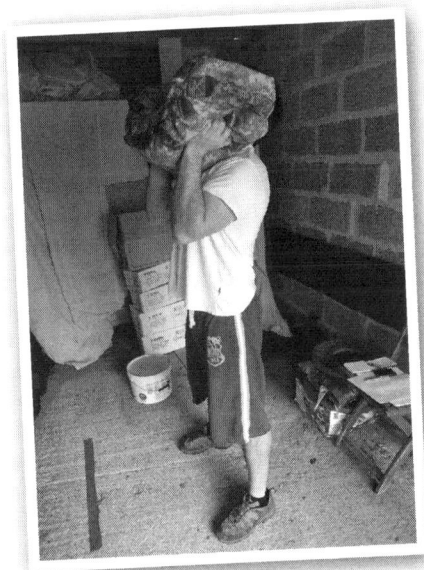

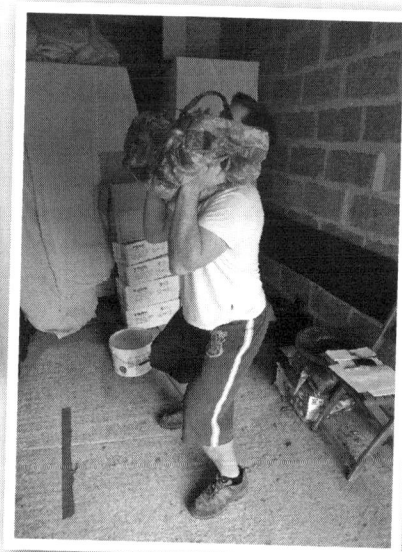

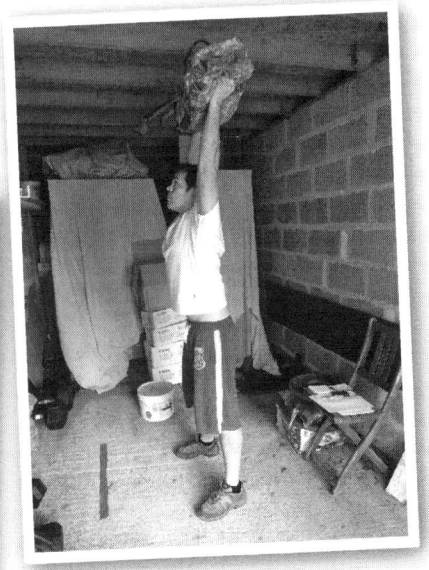

Sandbag Push Jerk

The Sandbag Push Jerk is an overhead press variation and the most powerful of all the overhead presses.

Technique

- Start with the sandbag at chest/shoulder height - as in a front squat
- Slightly bend the knees (dip) and then powerfully drive the sandbag overhead - using an extension through both the arms and legs (drive)
- Bend the knees to get back under the sandbag at the end of the movement (dip)
- DIP-DRIVE-DIP
- The arms should go to full extension
- The head should be slightly in front of the arms at this point of full extension
- Stay in neutral spine throughout
- Return to the starting position and repeat

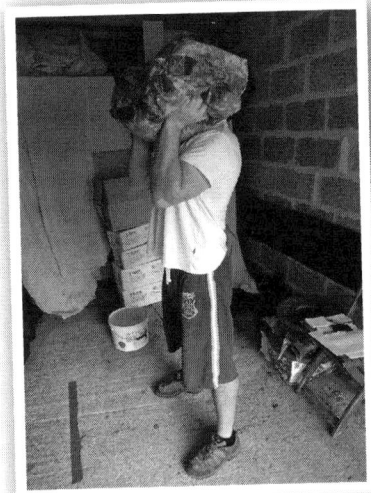

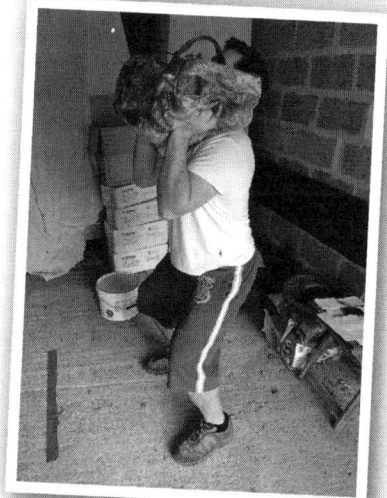

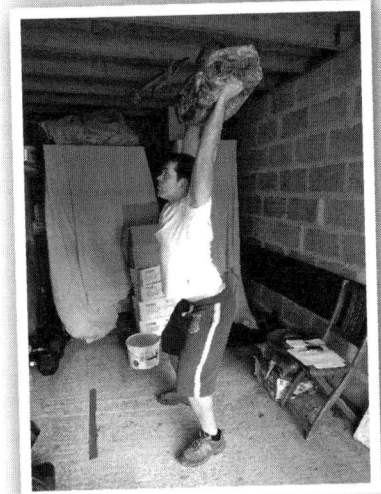

Sandbag Floor Press

The Sandbag Floor Press is our version of the bench press. It develops upper body strength and power, particularly in the chest and arms.

Technique

- Lie down on the ground with the sandbag in both hands, lying across your chest
- Push the sandbag straight upwards by extending your arms
- Arms should go to full extension
- Return the sandbag to the starting position and repeat

Variations

- Perform the exercise with a Hip Bridge (as pictured)

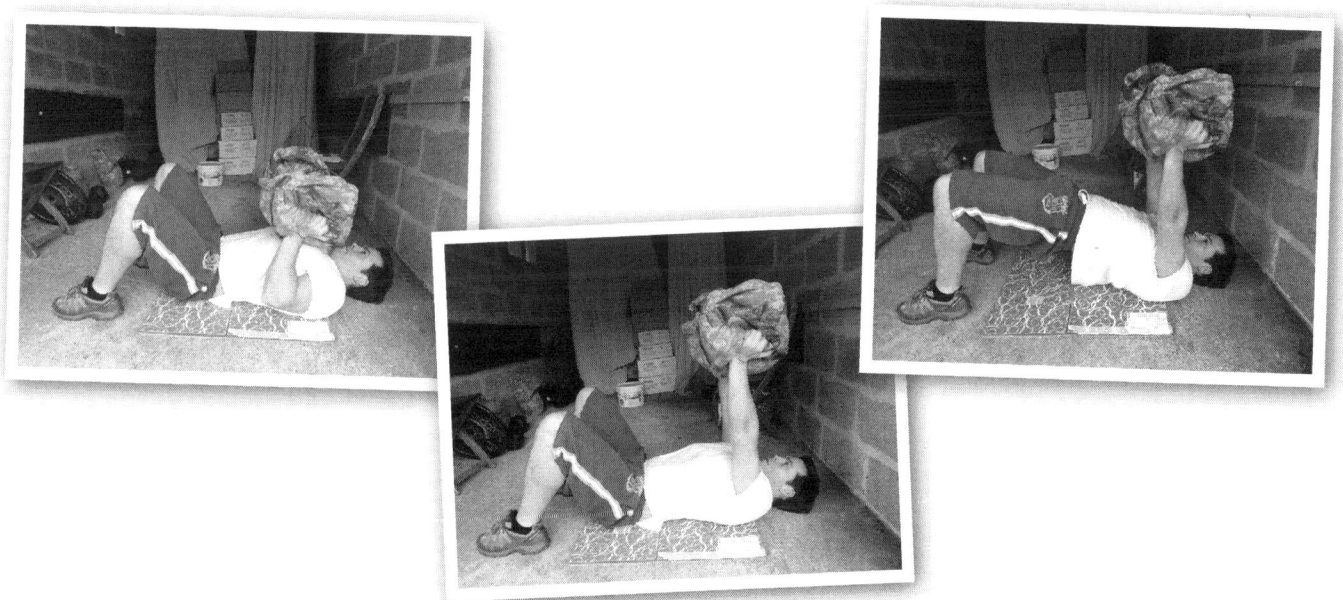

Sandbag Shoulder-to-Shoulder Press

The Sandbag Shoulder-to-Shoulder Press is an overhead press variation that is particularly challenging because the sandbag can be quite unstable in this position.

Technique

- Start with the sandbag resting on one shoulder with your hands underneath it
- Without additional help from the legs, press the sandbag upwards and above the head
- The arms should go to full extension
- The head should be slightly in front of the arms at this point of full extension
- Stay in neutral spine throughout
- Return to the opposite shoulder and repeat

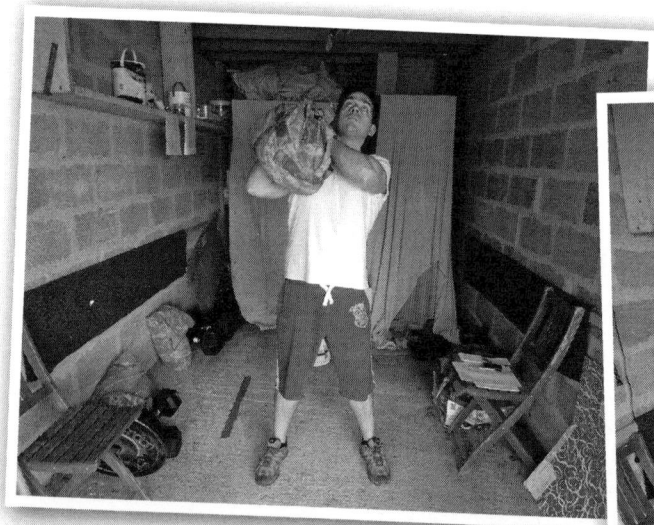

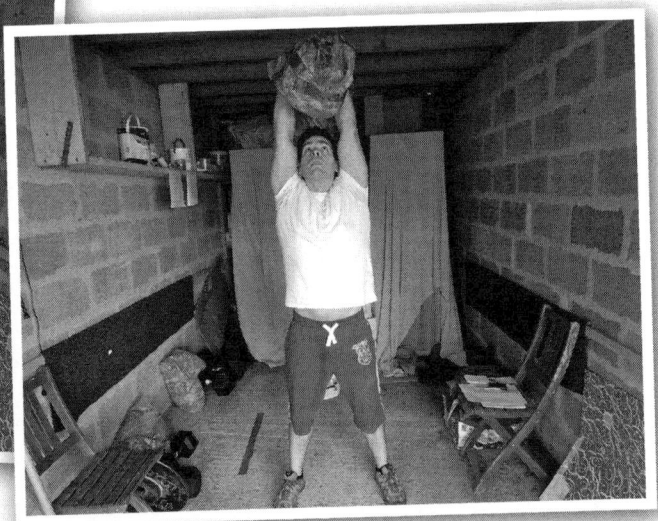

Press/Push Up

The Press Up aka the Push Up, correctly performed, builds upper body strength, endurance and core control. Maintaining a good Press Up position is virtually identical to the Plank exercise, except you need to maintain it under greater levels of stress (due to movement). For this reason, I think it is a great, multi-functional exercise.

Technique

- Hands are normally placed at shoulder width apart or slightly wider
- Lower your body all the way to the floor
- Chest, thighs and chin should touch the floor
- Push your body back upwards and return to the start position so that arms are straight
- Body stays tight throughout the movement
- Stay in neutral spine

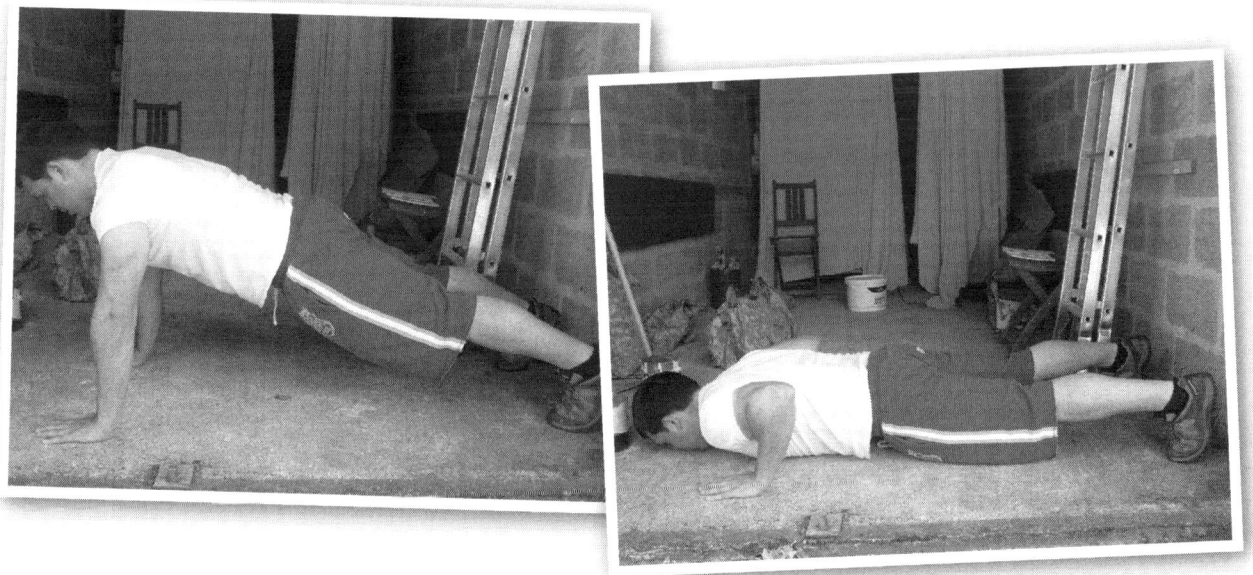

Press/Push Up

Variations

- Make it easier by performing the Press Up from the knees
- Experiment with different hand positions
- Increase the ROM by elevating yourself - I use 2 paint cans
- Add instability to the movement by performing it on Gymnastic Rings or similar equipment
- See 'T Press/Push Up'
- See 'Handstand Press/Push Up'

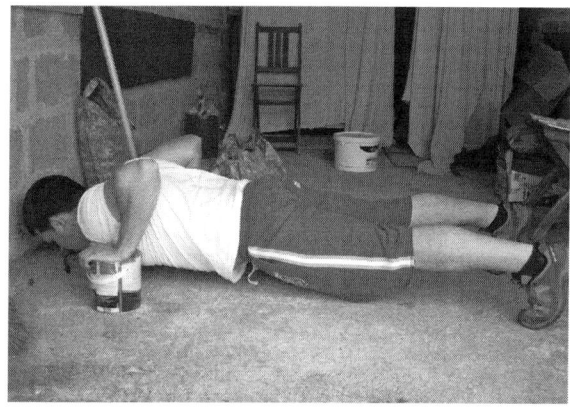

Increased ROM

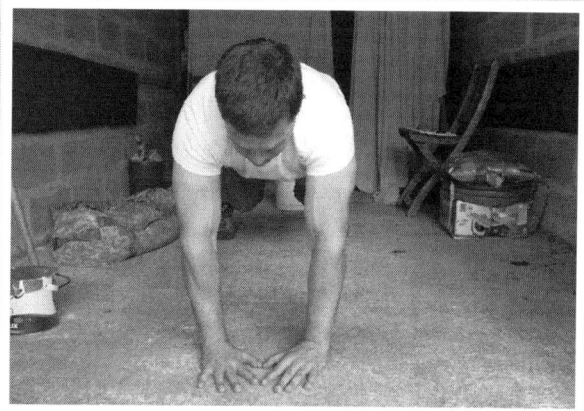

Narrow Grip

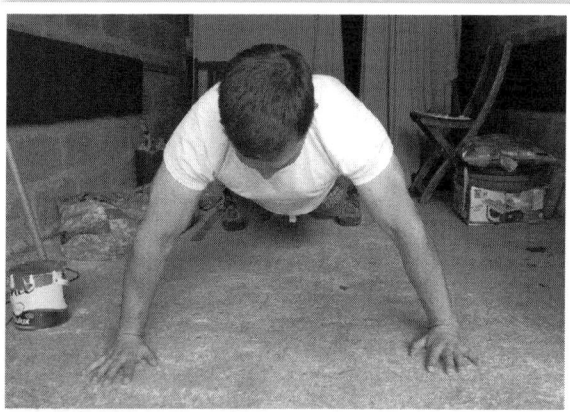

Wide Grip

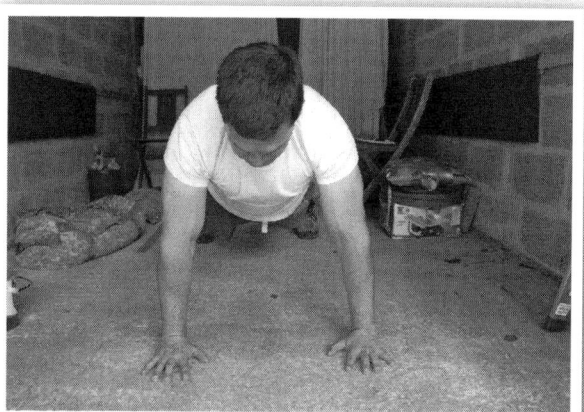

Regular Grip

Handstand Press/Push Up

The Handstand Press/Push Up is a serious upper body strength movement. It can be done anywhere and develops great shoulder and arm strength.

Technique

- Kick up against a solid wall or surface
- Hands should be placed around shoulder width apart
- Brace your core muscles throughout the movement
- Lower your head towards the ground by bending your arms
- Press yourself back upwards, returning to full arm extension

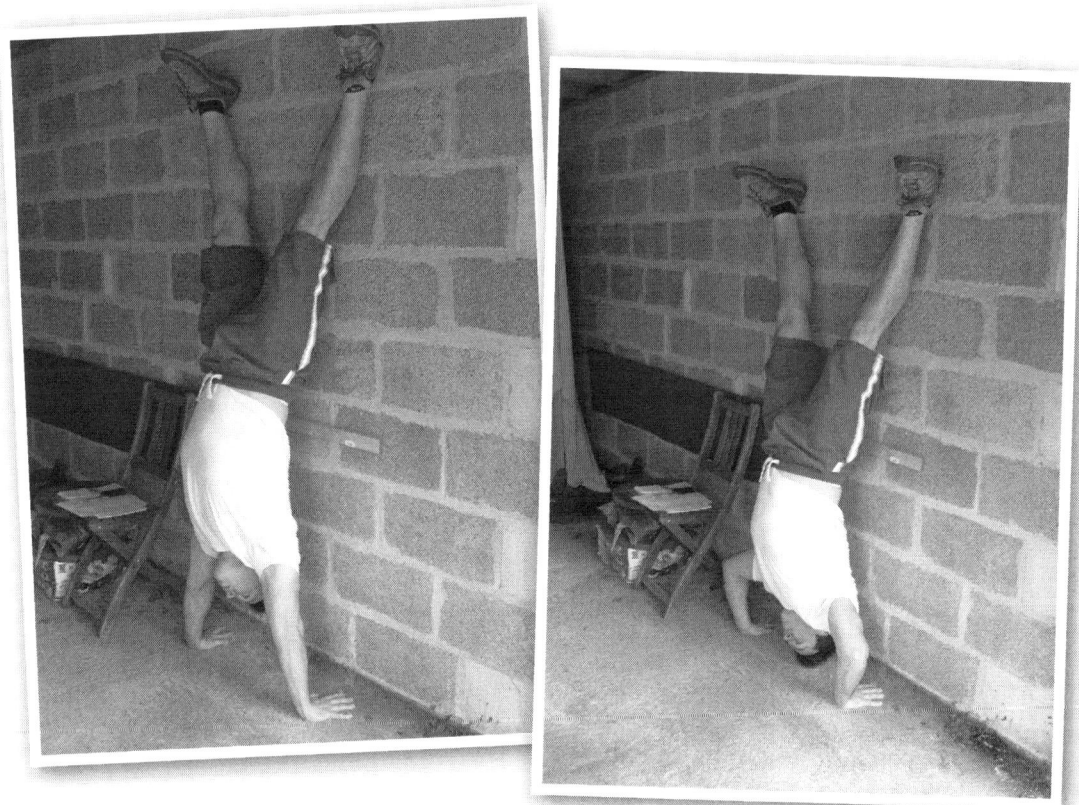

51

T Press/Push Up

The T Press/Push Up is a variation of the standard press/push up that encourages greater shoulder mobility and rotation.

Technique

- Hands are normally placed at shoulder width apart or slightly wider
- Lower your body all the way to the floor
- Chest, thighs and chin should touch the floor
- Push your body back upwards and begin to rotate your body outwards
- Lift one hand off the floor and, allowing your body to rotate, extend the arm upwards so that your arms and torso create a 'T' shape
- Stay in neutral spine throughout
- Return to the starting position and repeat on the other side

T Push Up

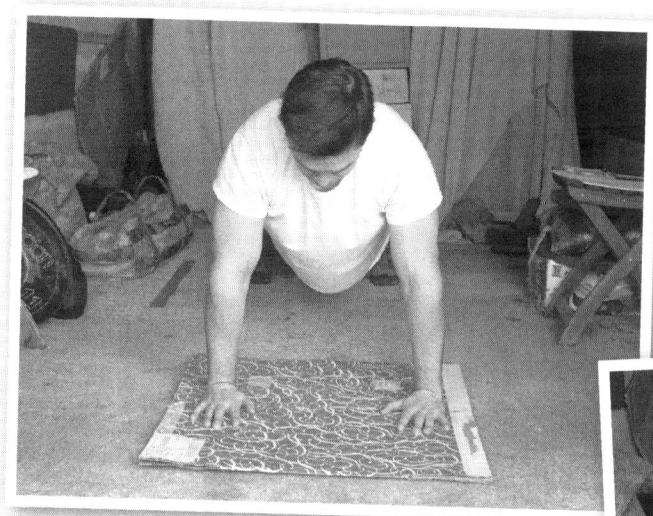

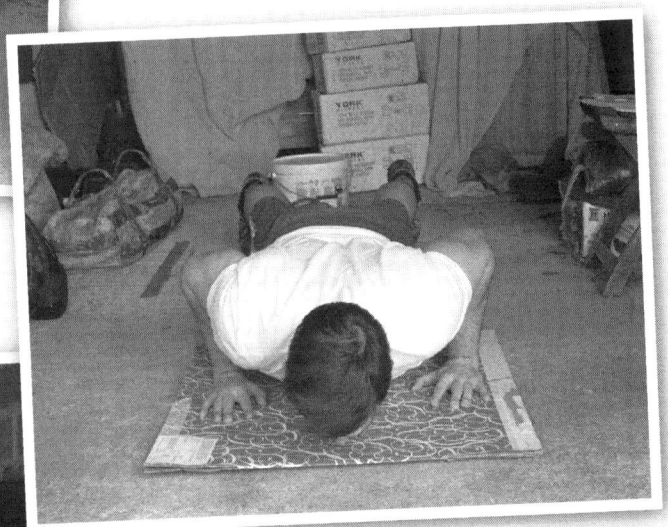

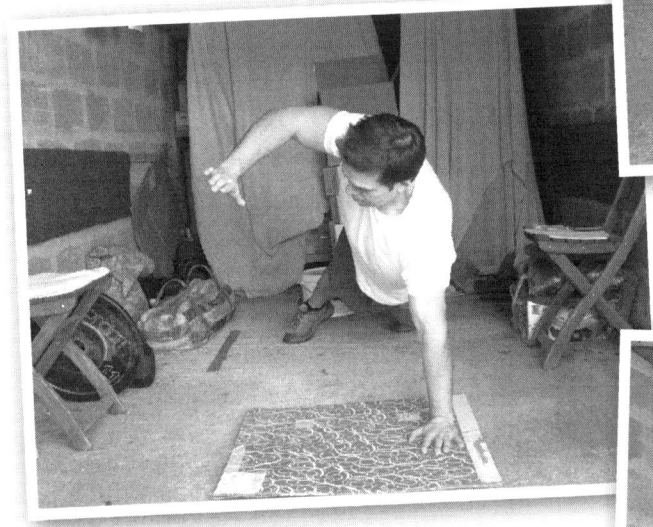

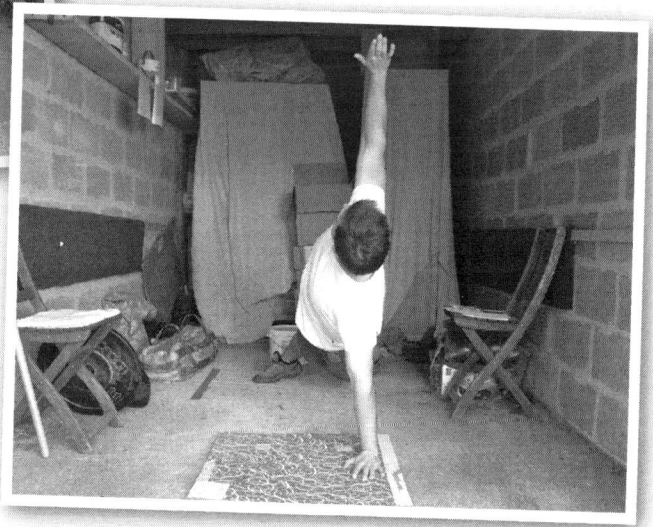

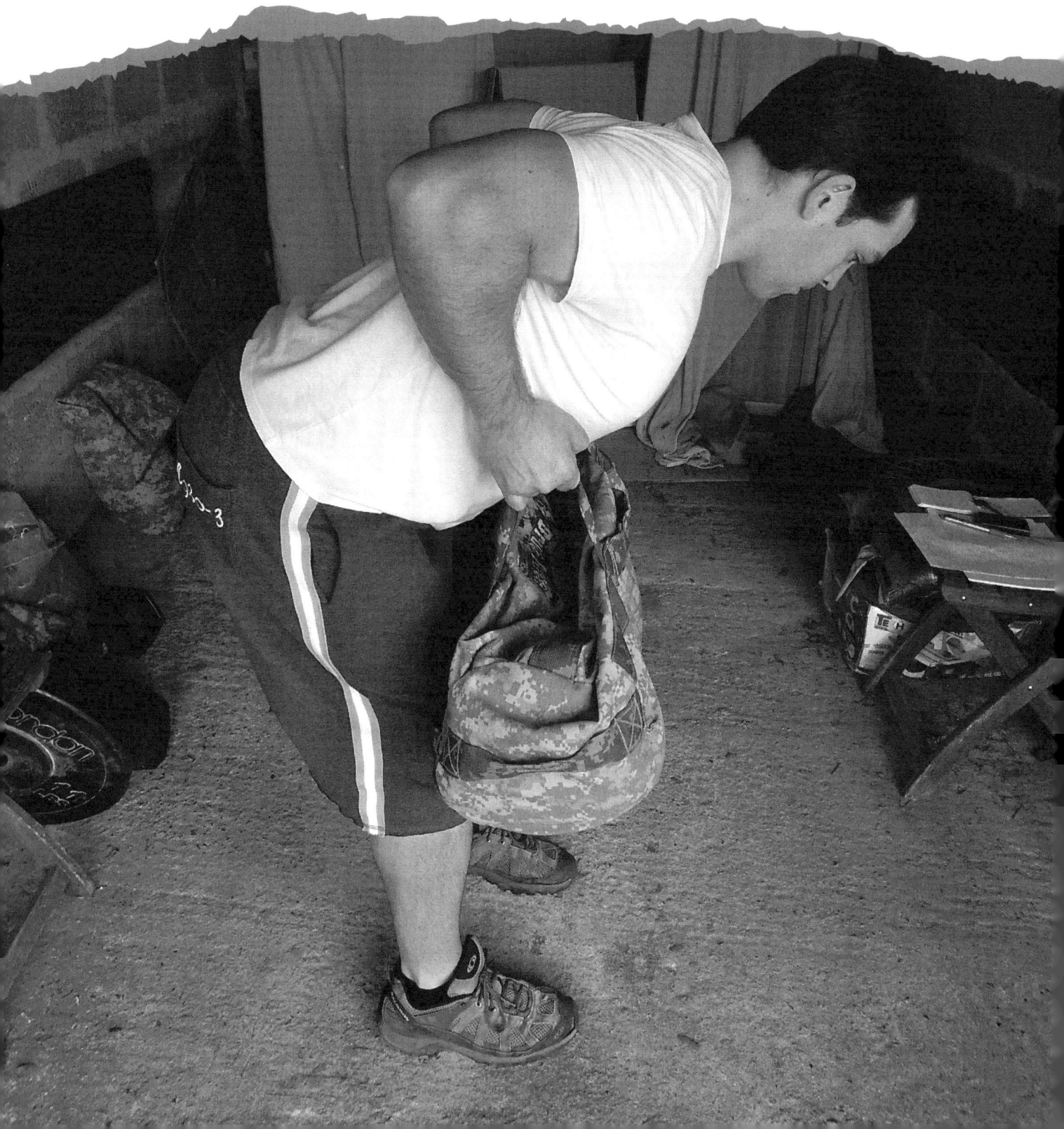

PULL

Sandbag Clean

The Sandbag Clean (and it's derivatives - the Sandbag Power Clean and the Sandbag Hang Clean) is one half of the Olympic Lift, the Clean and Jerk. It is also the standard technique for getting your sandbag, or any other weight, from the ground to chest height.

Technique

- Start as you would for a Sandbag Deadlift, with your feet slightly under the bag
- Set yourself ready
- Lift the bag from the ground and, as it gathers some momentum, explosively pull the bag upwards
- Try to use the power generated through your hips to do most of the work
- As the sandbag travels upwards prepare yourself to catch
- Do not throw the bag upwards, keep hold of it, but it should become almost weightless
- Catch the bag with a Zercher grip or at either end of the sandbag
- Descend into a Squat
- Return back to standing as though coming out of a Sandbag Front Squat
- Return the bag to the ground in a fluid movement

Variations

- A Sandbag Power Clean is the same except you do not squat as part of the lift
- A Sandbag Hang Clean is the same except the sandbag is pulled from mid thigh instead of from the ground

Sandbag Clean

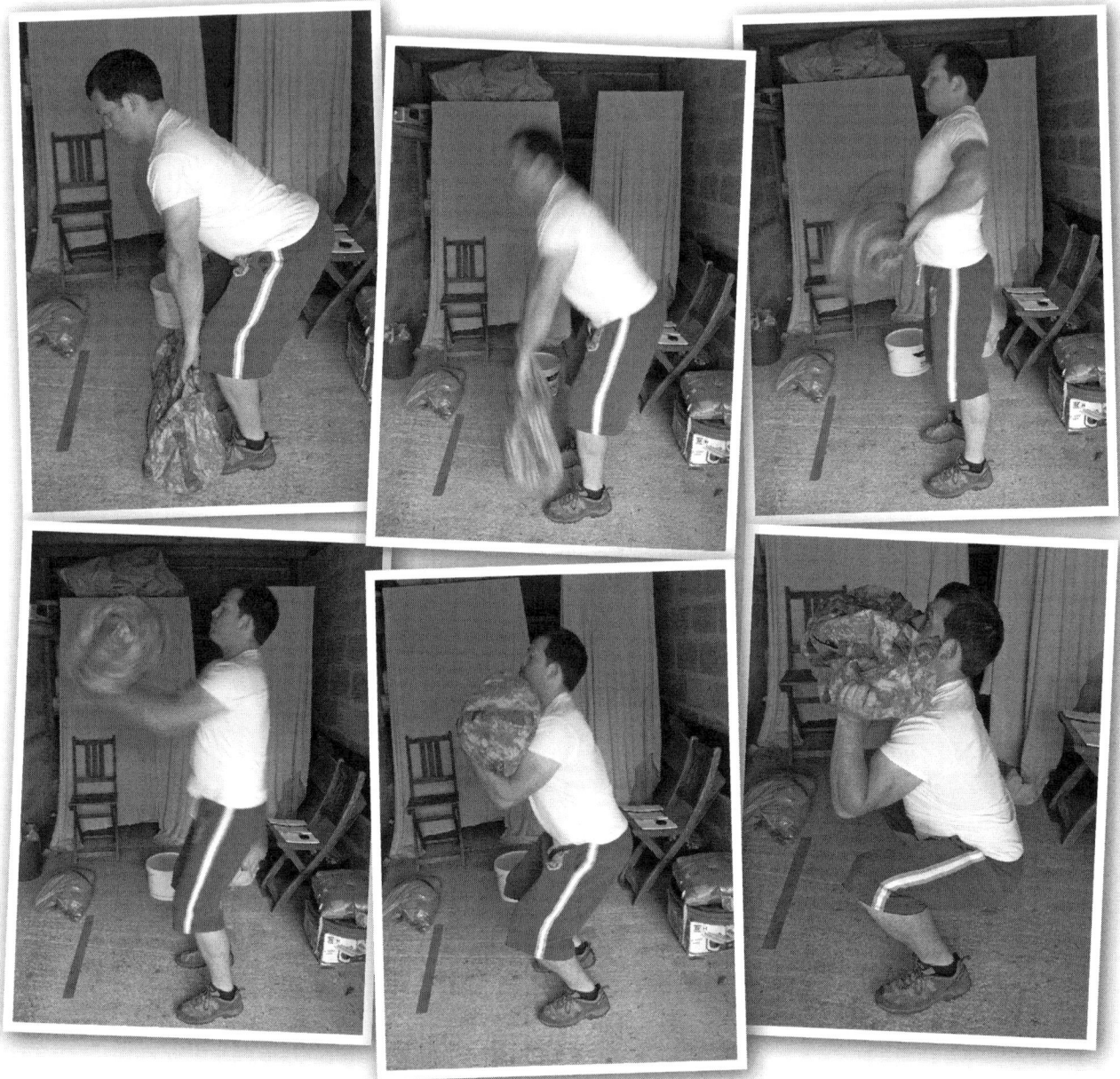

Sandbag High Pull

The Sandbag High Pull is a progression exercise for the Sandbag Clean and also develops power in the posterior chain.

Technique

- Stand over the sandbag, as if you are going to Deadlift or Clean it
- Take the weight
- Explode powerfully upwards - extending the hips fully and pulling the weight quickly up to chest/chin height
- Try to use the power generated through your hips to do most of the work
- The elbows should be high at the top of the movement
- Open the chest out at the top of the movement
- Return the sandbag to the floor and repeat

Variations

- Single-arm High Pulls

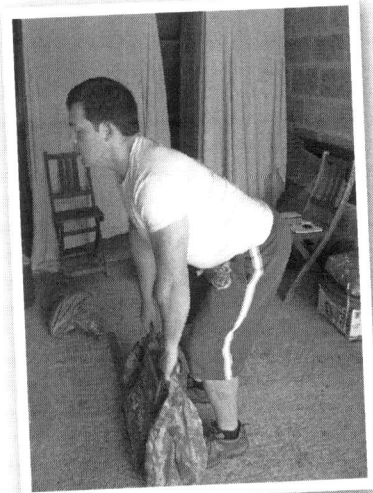

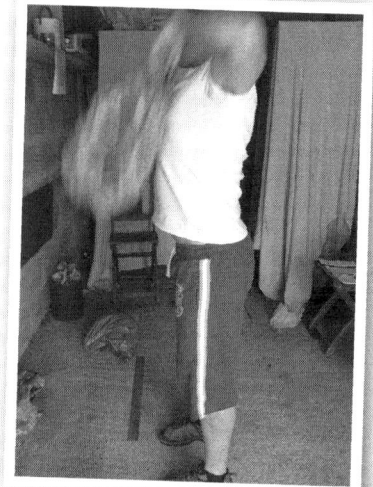

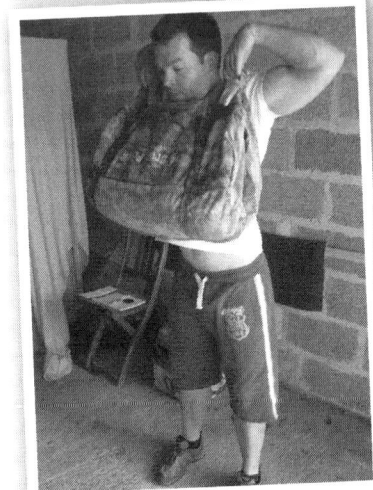

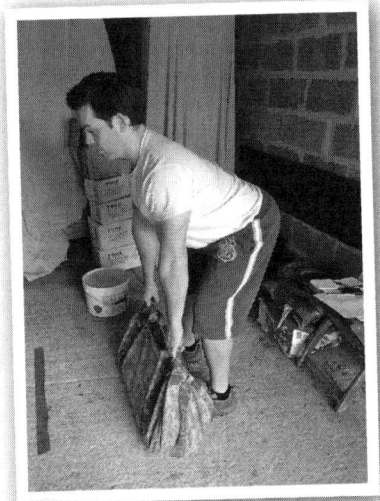

Sandbag Snatch

The Sandbag Snatch is similar to the Sandbag High Pull but differs in that the sandbag travels overhead. This makes the snatch a great power movement.

Technique

- Stand over the sandbag, as if you are going to Deadlift or Clean it
- Take the weight
- Explode powerfully upwards - extending the hips fully and pulling the weight quickly up to chest/chin height
- Try to use the power generated through your hips to do most of the work
- The elbows should be high throughout the movement
- As the sandbag reaches chest height, drop yourself downwards
- Fully extend you arms overhead
- Return the sandbag to the floor and repeat

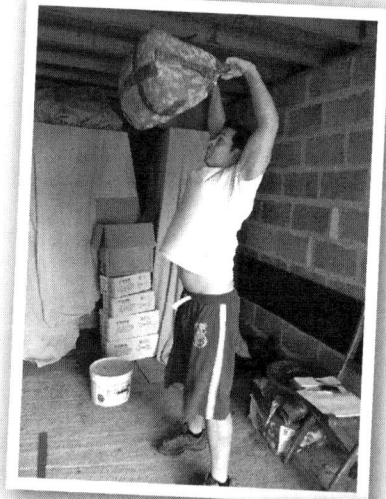
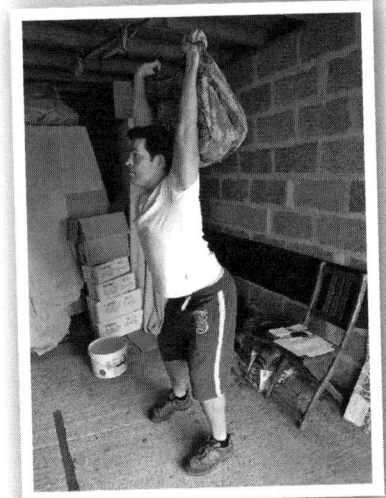

Sandbag Bent Over Row

The Sandbag Bent Over Row is designed to develop strength and power in the back. It also puts a great demand on your lower back and core muscles.

Technique

- Hold your sandbag in both hands
- Lean forward until your torso is at at least 45°, knees should be slightly bent
- Pull the sandbag in towards your body
- Return to the start position and repeat
- Make sure you maintain a good neutral spine position throughout

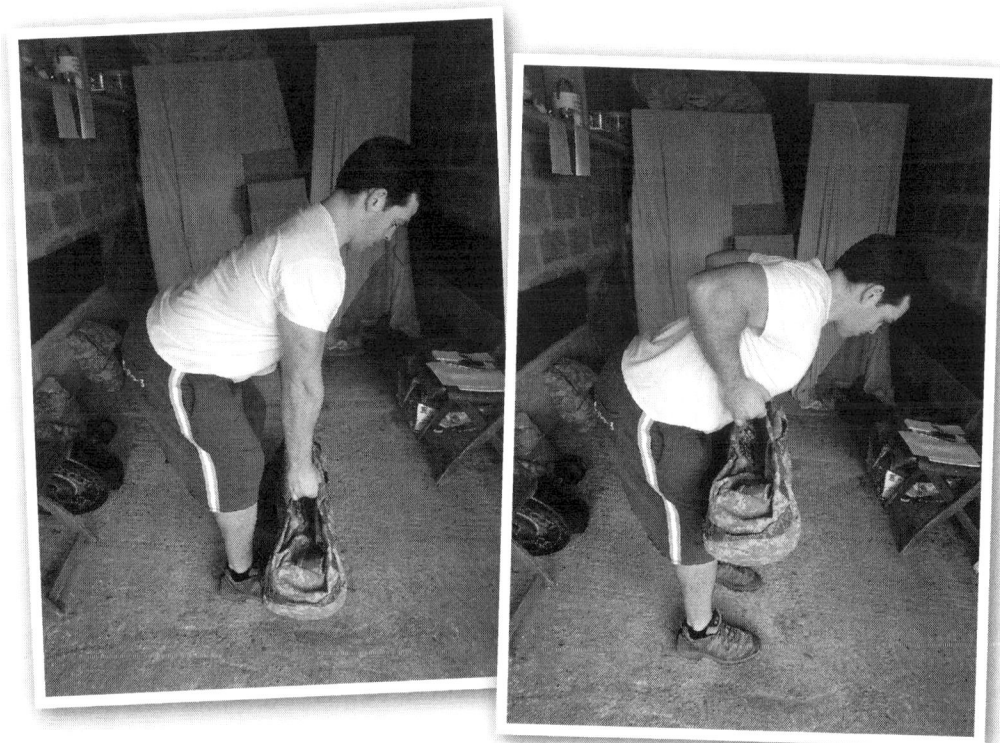

Sandbag Shouldering

Sandbag Shouldering is one of those exercises that looks deceptively easy. This move will help you to develop brute strength and power. A great exercise for contact sportspeople too.

Technique

- Take hold of the sandbag in any way that you can
- Powerfully lift the sandbag up onto your shoulder
- Return the sandbag back to the ground and repeat on the opposite side
- Aim to maintain good clean technique throughout

Sandbag Shouldering

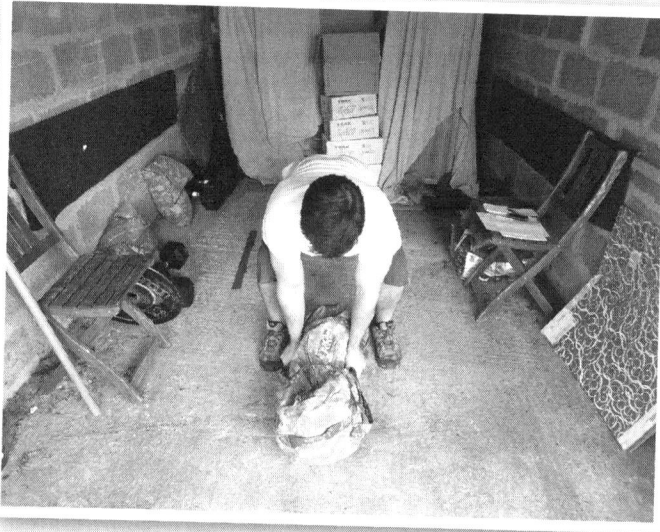

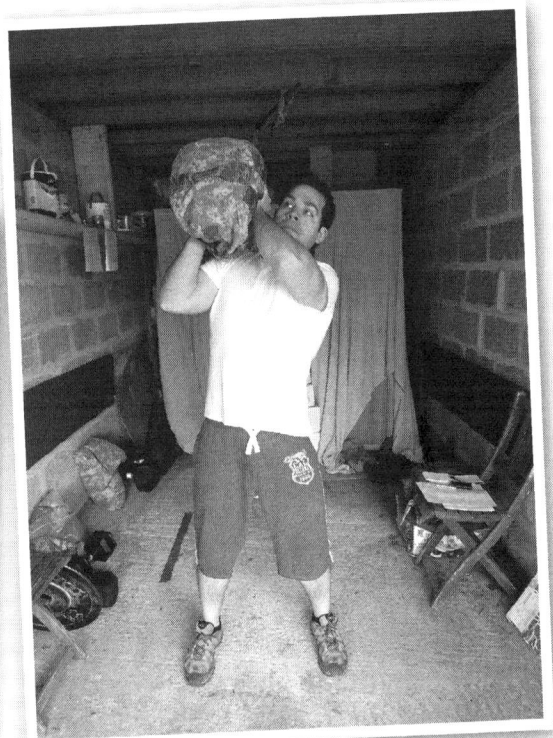

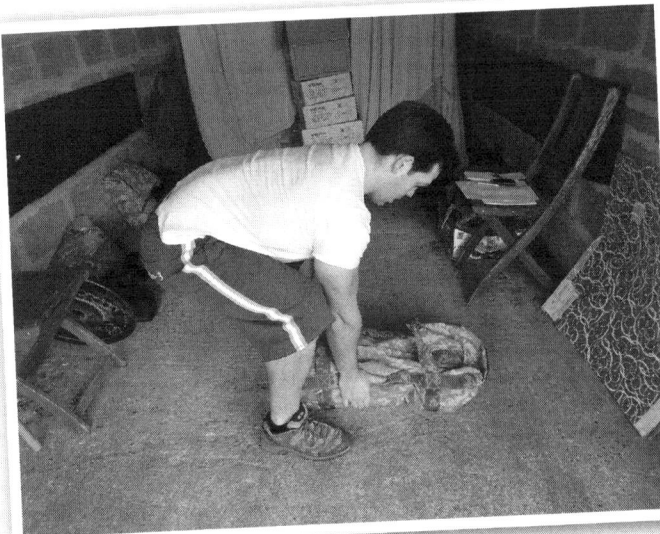

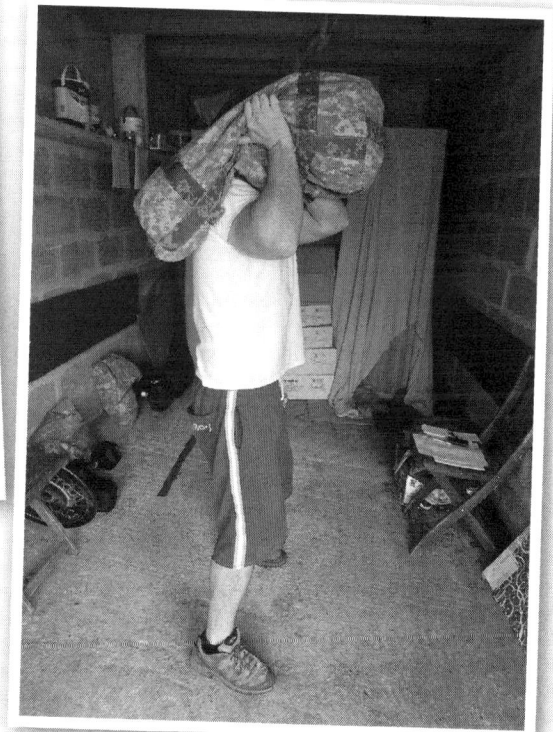

Pull Ups

The Pull Up is one of our top bodyweight conditioning exercises. A great exercise for building upper body pulling strength and the ultimate in function for anyone who wants to get good at climbing or pulling their body over obstacles.

Technique

- Hang from a bar (or anything you can e.g. Gymnastic Rings, TRX, a tree branch, a door frame)
- Pull your body upwards until your chin is above the bar/your hands
- Return to full hang/full extension through the elbow and shoulder before repeating

Variations

- 'Kipping' Pull Ups (see below)
- Inverted Row (or Australian Pull Up)
- Jumping Pull Ups - use a small jump to aid the pull
- Add weight to make the exercise harder
- See 'Gorilla Pull Ups'
- See 'L Pull Ups'

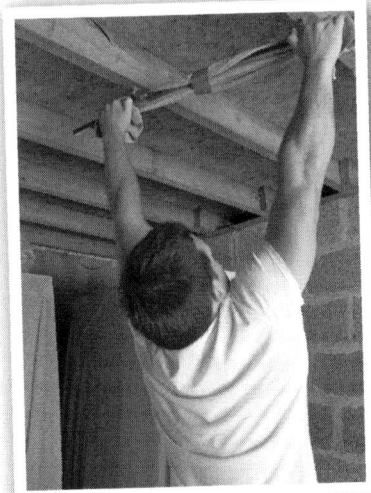

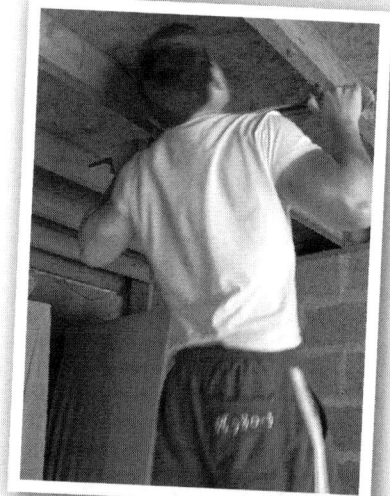

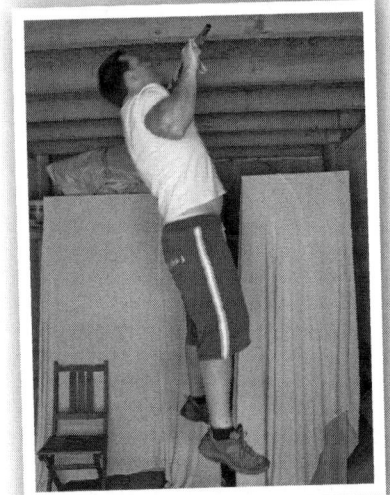

Pull Ups

"To kip, or not to kip"

Kipping is a style of pull up that has been made popular by Crossfit. It involves aiding the upper body strength by adding additional body movement and generating some dynamic power. Many call this cheating, but really it is just a different variation of the movement and will accomplish slightly different ends. While both are great exercises for developing pulling strength - the kipping pull up is more effective for power and agility while the strict pull up is a better pure strength exercise. I recommend doing both.

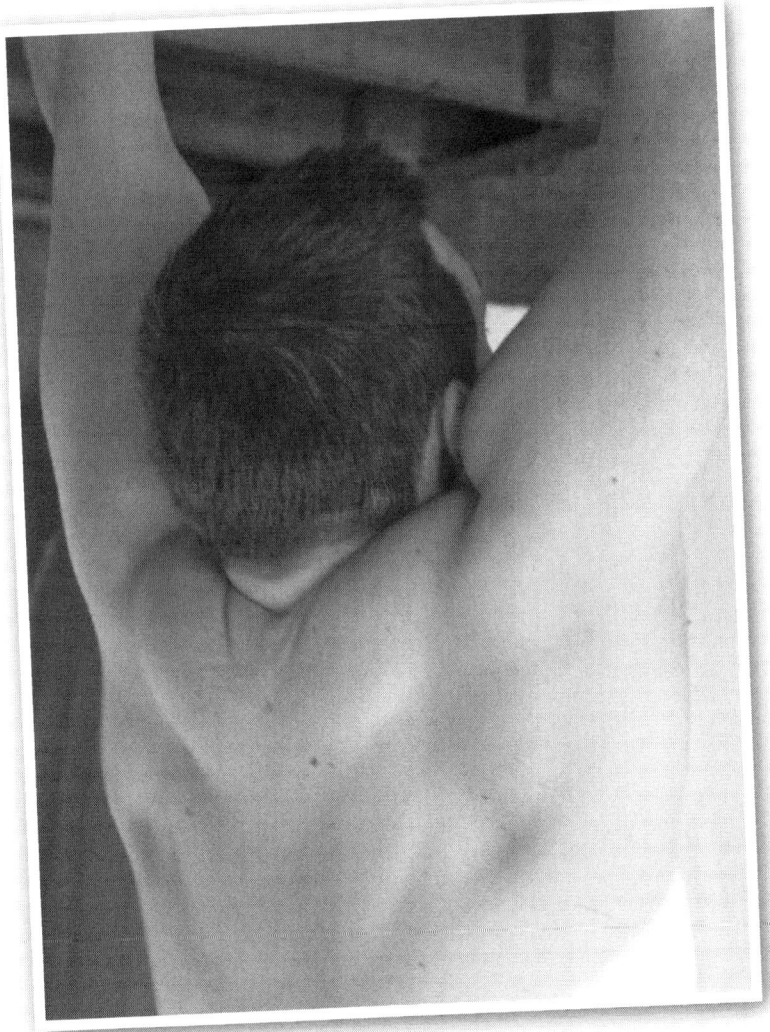

Gorilla Pull Ups

A pull up variation, the Gorilla Pull Up is a combination of both pull up and knee raise. A great exercise if you're short on time as you can develop upper body strength and core strength at the same time.

Technique

- Hang from a bar (or anything you can e.g. Gymnastic Rings, TRX, a tree branch, a door frame)
- As you pull your body upwards, bring your knees up towards your chest
- Your knees should reach chest height at the very top of the pull up
- Return to full hang/full extension through the elbow and shoulder before repeating

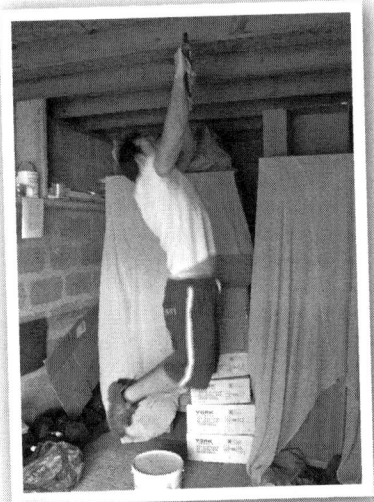

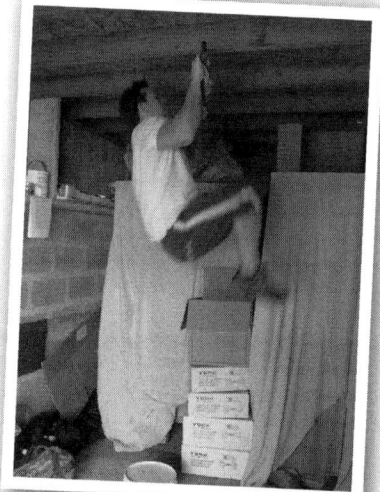

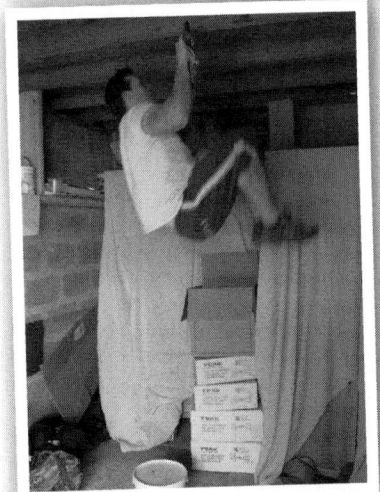

L Pull Ups

The L Pull Up is another pull up variation that places extra stress on the core muscles - making it very versatile. Easily the toughest pull up variation in this guide.

Technique

- Hang from a bar (or anything you can e.g. Gymnastic Rings, TRX, a tree branch, a door frame)
- Lift your straight legs out towards the front of your body
- Keeping your legs extended, pull your body upwards until your chin is above the bar/your hands
- Return to full hang/full extension through the elbow and shoulder before repeating
- Aim to keep legs straight throughout the exercise

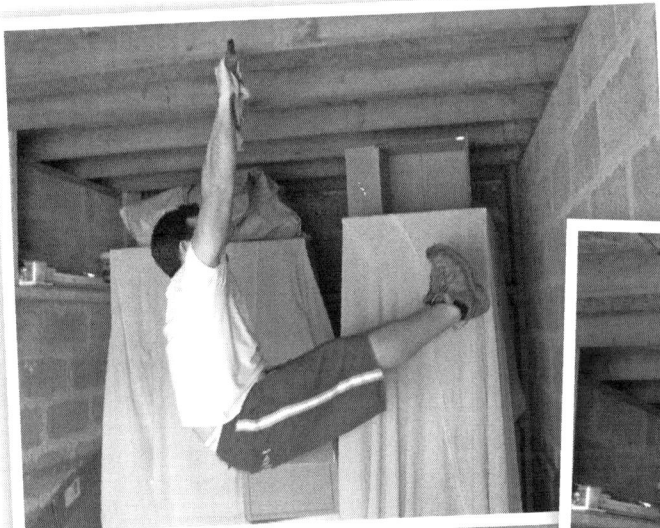

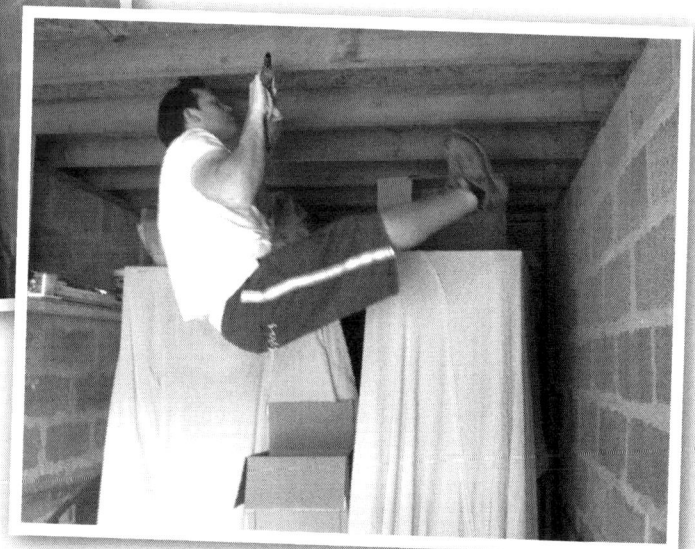

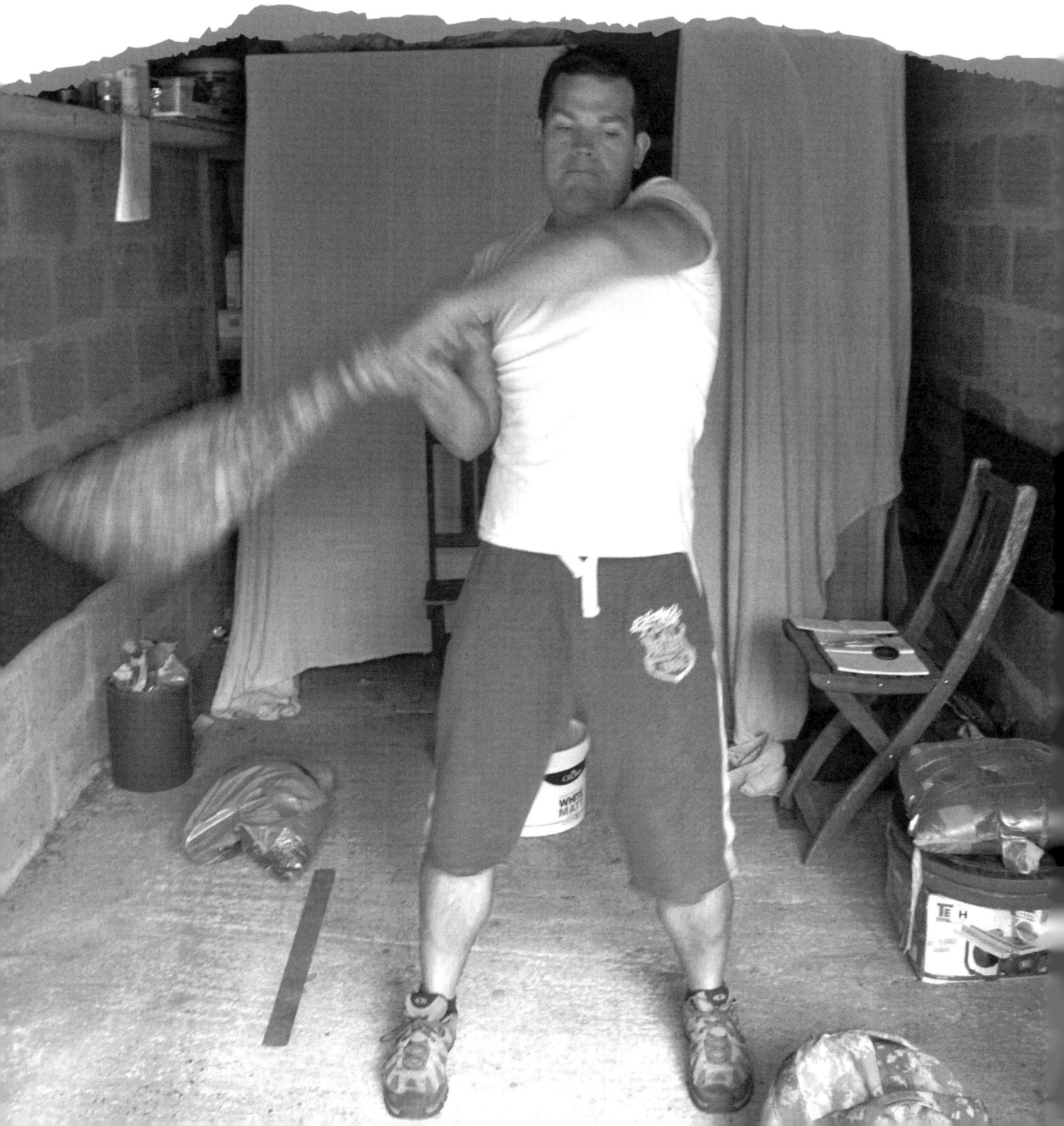

CORE

Sandbag Round-the-World

The inclusion of the Sandbag Round-the-World in this training guide is partly to develop rotational power, and also to aid any flexibility issues through the core and shoulders. It has a great transference into athletic ability and will build high levels of power and agility. Plus, it's just plain fun to swing something around your head.

Technique

- You can use either a homemade 'Tornado Ball' or one of your filler bags from your Brute Force Sandbag
- Take hold of the bag in two hands
- Swing the bag around your body while maintaining a stable base - feet should be shoulder width apart and remain fixed
- Be sure to extend your arms fully in front of the body
- Repeat in each direction

Variations

- Try single-handed Round-the-Worlds
- Practice swinging the sandbag in different directions

Sandbag Round-the-World

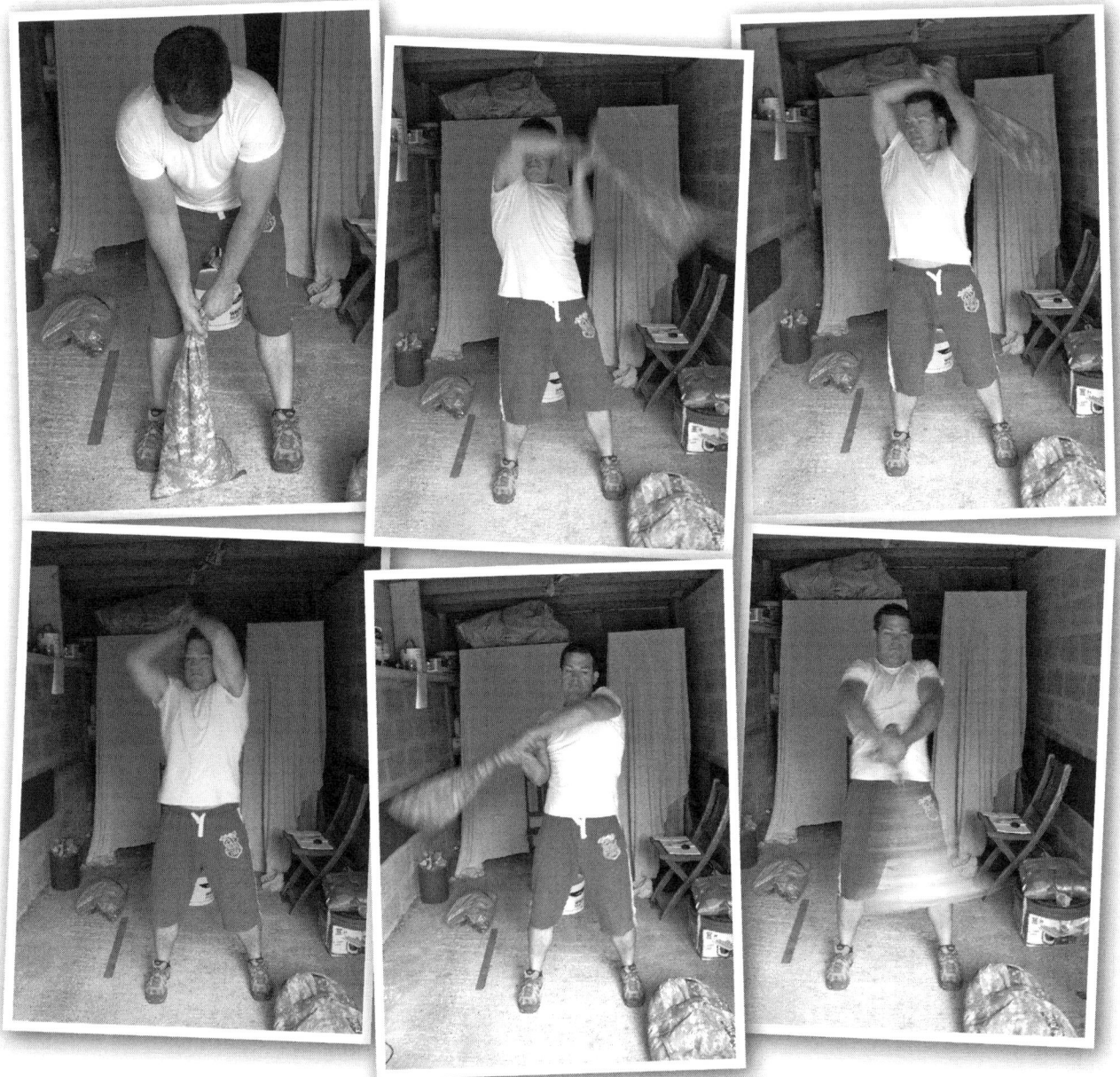

Sandbag Windmill

The Sandbag Windmill is the ultimate exercise for core strength and mobility. It's also an excellent movement for shoulder stability.

Technique

- Lift your sandbag up to shoulder height and hold it in one hand
- Turn your feet at 45° to the working arm
- Press the sandbag overhead and keep the arm straight for the remainder of the exercise
- Push your hip out to the side and reach down towards the floor
- Look up towards the sandbag and allow the shoulder to rotate is necessary
- The working arm MUST stay fully extended

Variations

- See 'Sandbag Bent Press'

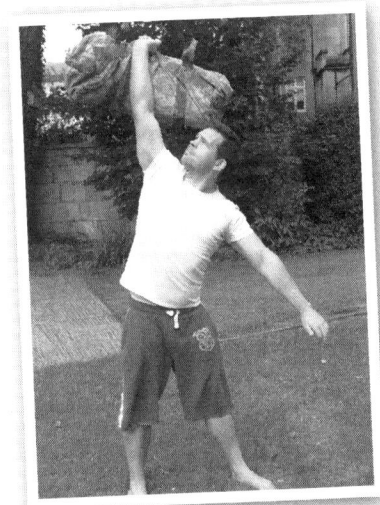

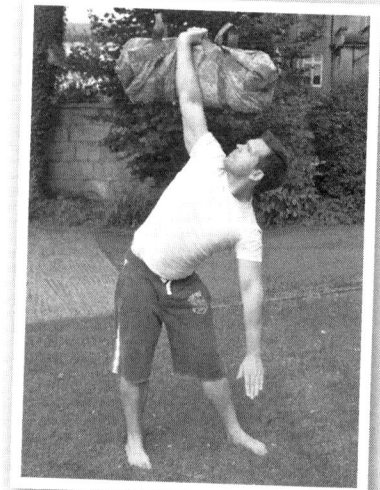

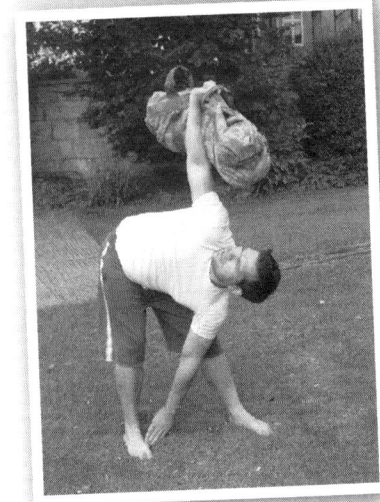

Sandbag Bent Press

The Sandbag Bent Press is a windmill variation that also builds upper body pressing strength and power.

Technique

- Lift your sandbag up to shoulder height and hold it in one hand
- Turn your feet at 45° to the working arm
- Push your hip out to the side
- Reach down towards the ground as you press the sandbag upwards
- Look up towards the sandbag and allow the shoulder to rotate is necessary
- Aim to touch the ground as the working arm fully extends
- Return to the start position and repeat

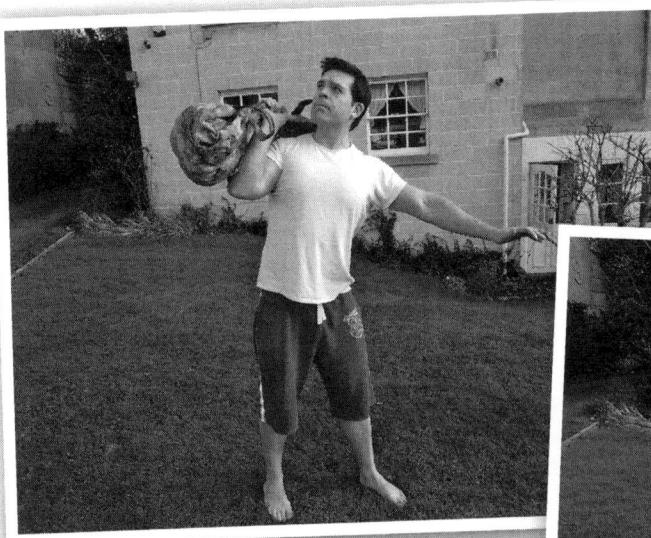

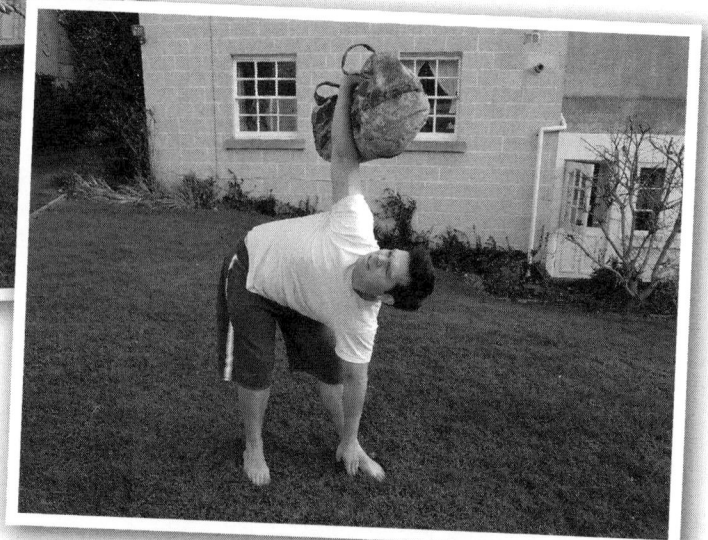

Sandbag Good Morning

The Sandbag Good Morning is great for strengthening hamstrings and the lower back. It is also the perfect exercise to accompany the deadlift.

Technique

- Start with the sandbag across your shoulder
- Set your back into a good neutral spine position
- Push your hips backwards and lean forwards
- Allow your hamstrings to lengthen as you lean forwards
- Keep the back straight throughout
- Return to full hip extension between repetitions

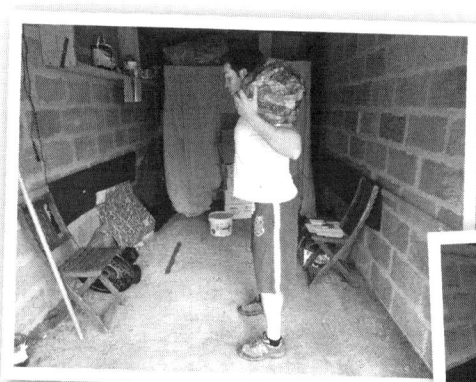

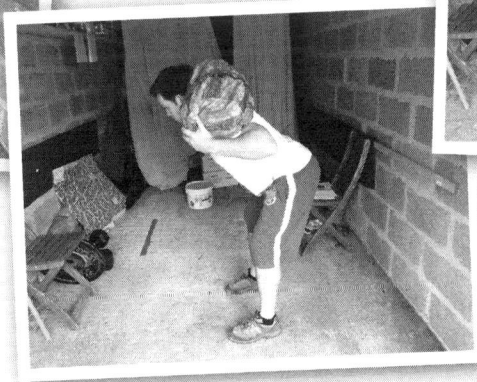

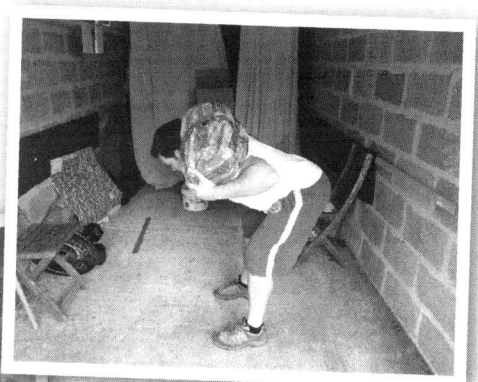

Sit Up

The Sit Up has a particularly bad reputation and has largely been replaced by the far inferior Crunch in recent times. The ability to actually sit up is important so I see no reason to omit it from any exercise programme - just pay attention to neutral spine and correct head position and you'll have no problems.

Technique

- Sit on the floor with your knees bent at around 90 degrees
- Fix your feet under your sandbag
- Keeping the chest and head high, sit upwards until your body is fully upright
- Return back to the floor - your head and shoulders should touch down between repetitions
- Use a mat if you need to - I use some cardboard

Variations

- Make the exercise harder by adding additional weight

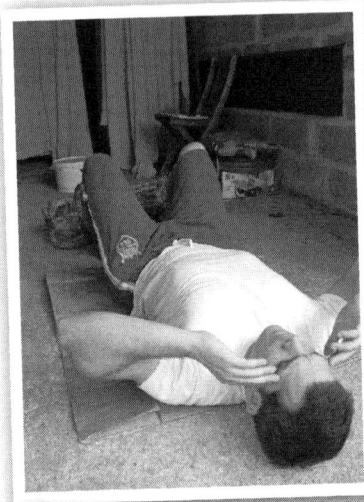
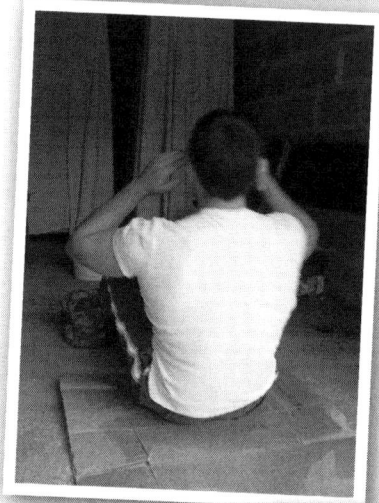
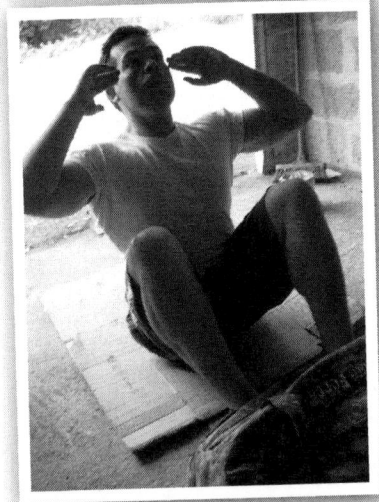

Knees-to-Elbows

Knees-to-Elbows are a great core exercise that will also do wonders for your agility and grip strength. Work hard to get your knees all the way up to your elbows and you'll really notice the difference in your midsection strength.

Technique

- Hang from a bar (or anything you can e.g. Gymnastic Rings, TRX, or a tree branch)
- Bring your knees up to the tips of your elbows
- This can be done with straight arms or a slight bend at the elbow - find out what works for you
- Return to a full hang/full extension through the elbow and shoulder before repeating

Variations

- You can make this exercise easier by performing a Hanging Knee Raise - where the knees are raised to waist height
- See 'Toes-to-Bar'
- See 'Hanging Leg Raises'

Knees-to-Elbows

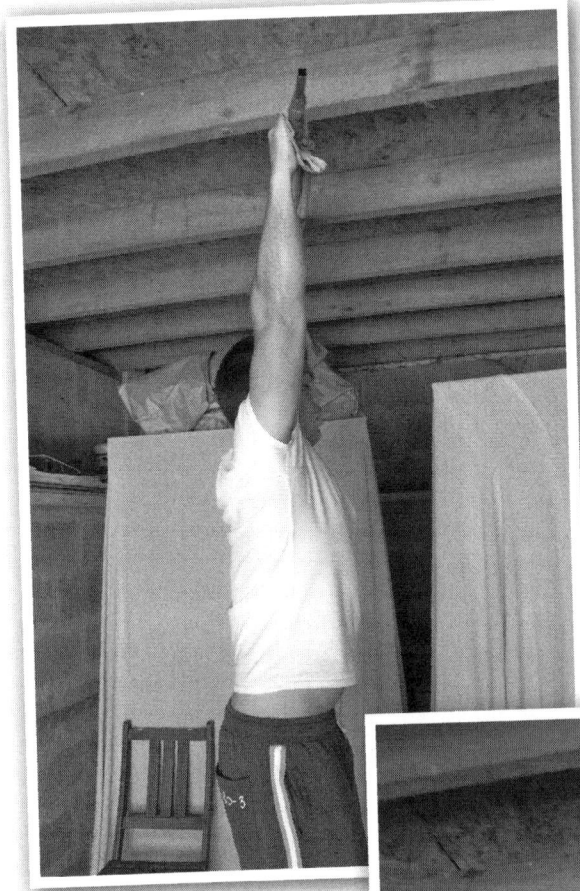

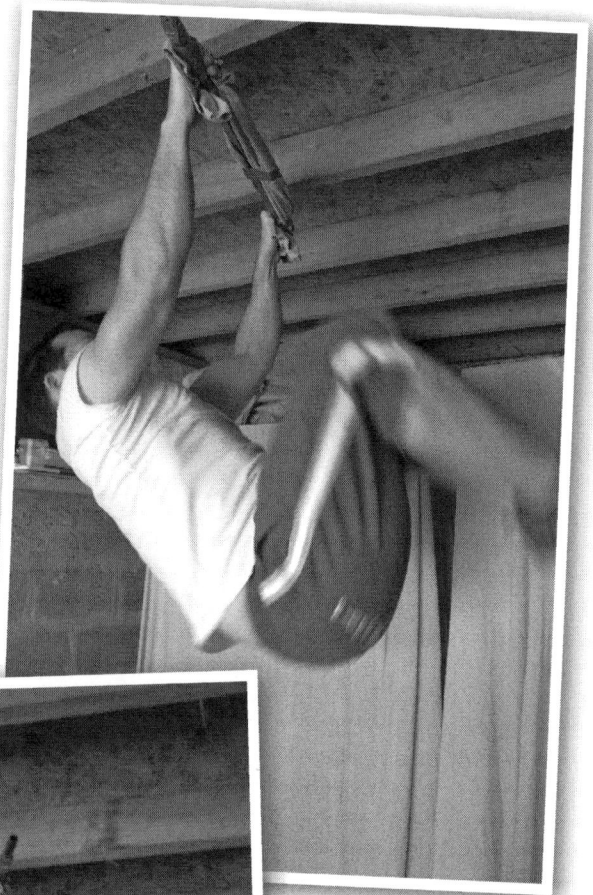

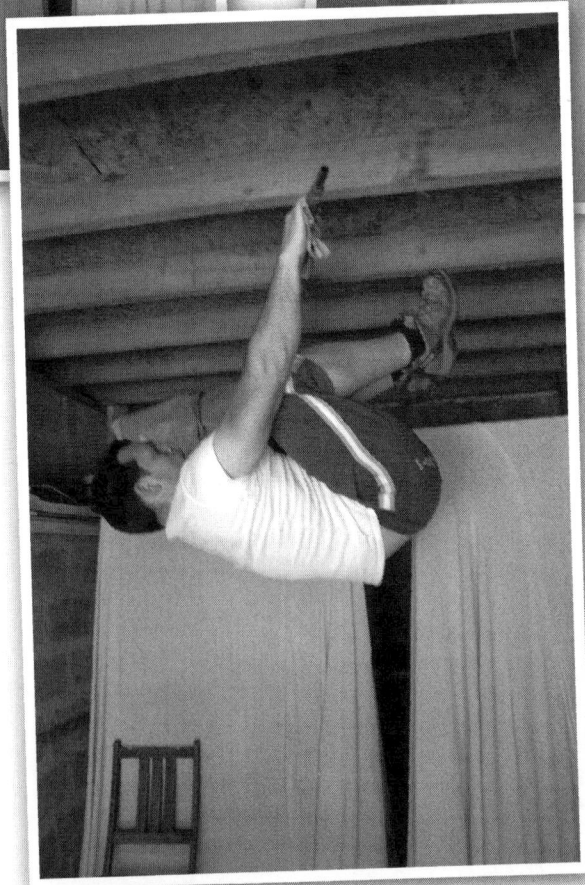

Toes-to-Bar

Toes-to-Bar are an advanced progression of Knee-to-Elbows and require a good degree of core and grip strength.

Technique

- Hang from a bar (or anything you can e.g. Gymnastic Rings, TRX, a tree branch)
- Bring your toes up to touch the bar
- This can be done with straight arms or a slight bend at the elbow - find out what works for you
- Return to a full hang/full extension through the elbow and shoulder before repeating
- I'm pictured with bent knees (due to space restrictions) but you should aim to do it with straight legs if possible

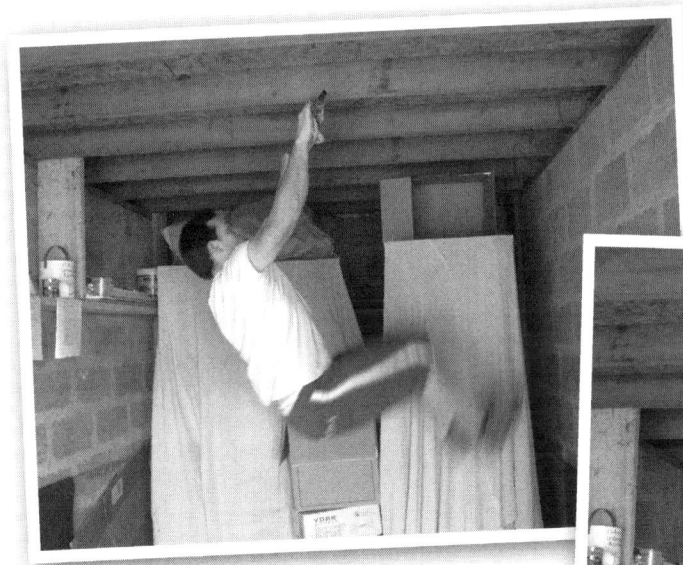

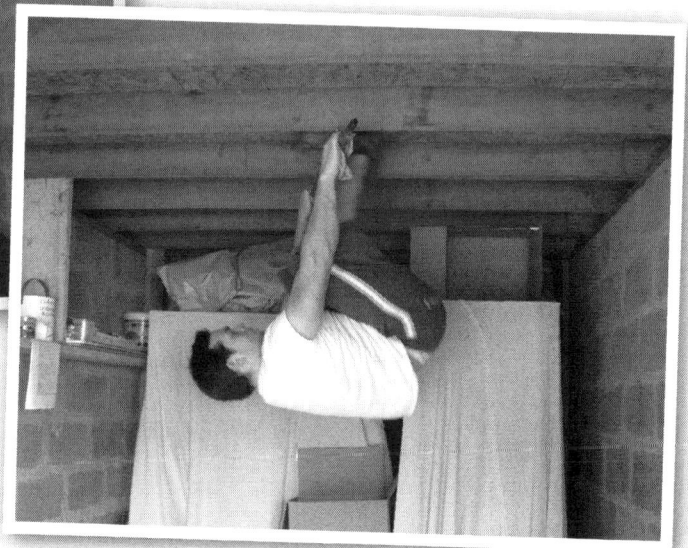

Hanging Leg Raise

The Hanging Leg Raise is a progression from knees-to-elbows. Great for developing core and hip flexor strength and grip.

Technique

- Hang from a bar (or anything you can e.g. Gymnastic Rings, TRX, a tree branch)
- Lift your straight legs upwards - aim for at least 90°
- Try to keep your arms straight throughout the exercise
- Return to a full hang/full extension through the hip before repeating

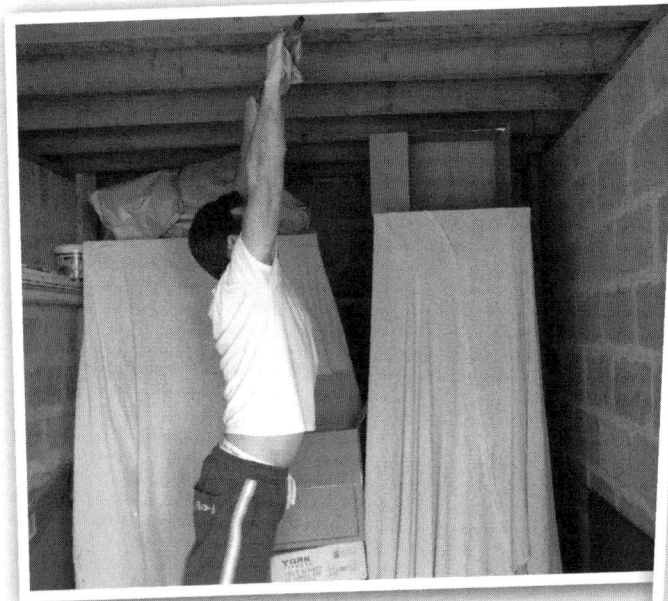

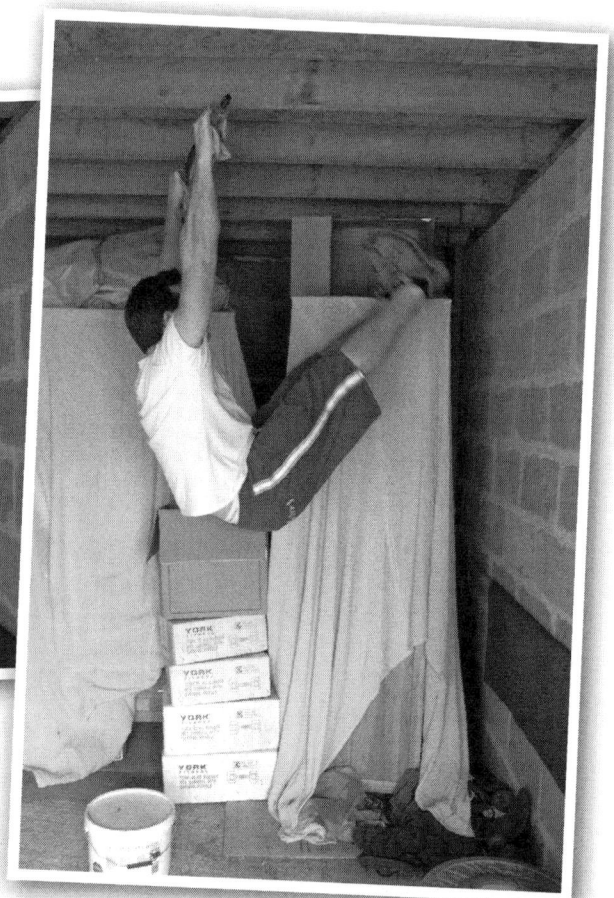

Plank

The Plank builds static strength, primarily in the core muscles. Another exercise that can be done anywhere.

How To

- Lie face down on the ground
- Set your forearms under your shoulders
- Lift yourself upwards so that you are supported on just forearms and the balls of your feet
- Keep your abdominal muscles braced throughout the exercise
- Remember to breathe

Variations

- You can make the exercise easier by performing from the knees
- Try single leg variations

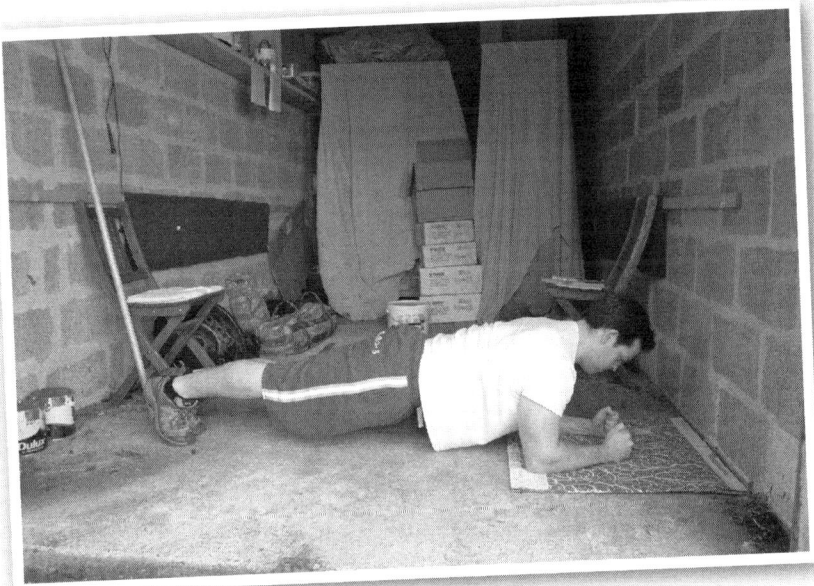

Lower Back Raise

A useful strengthening exercise for the lower back.

Technique

- Lie face down on the ground
- Keeping your hips and feet in contact with the ground, lift your head and chest upwards
- Aim to keep your head in a neutral position
- Keep the movement smooth

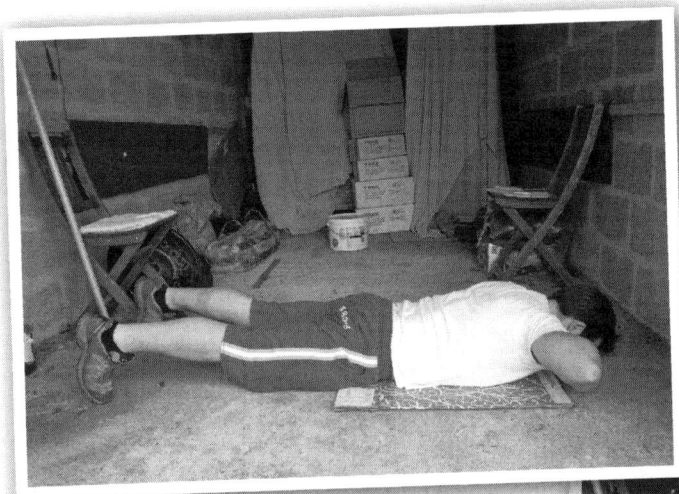

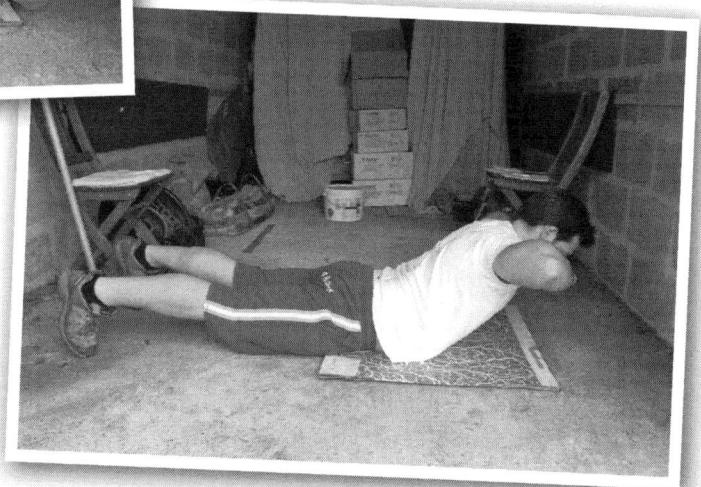

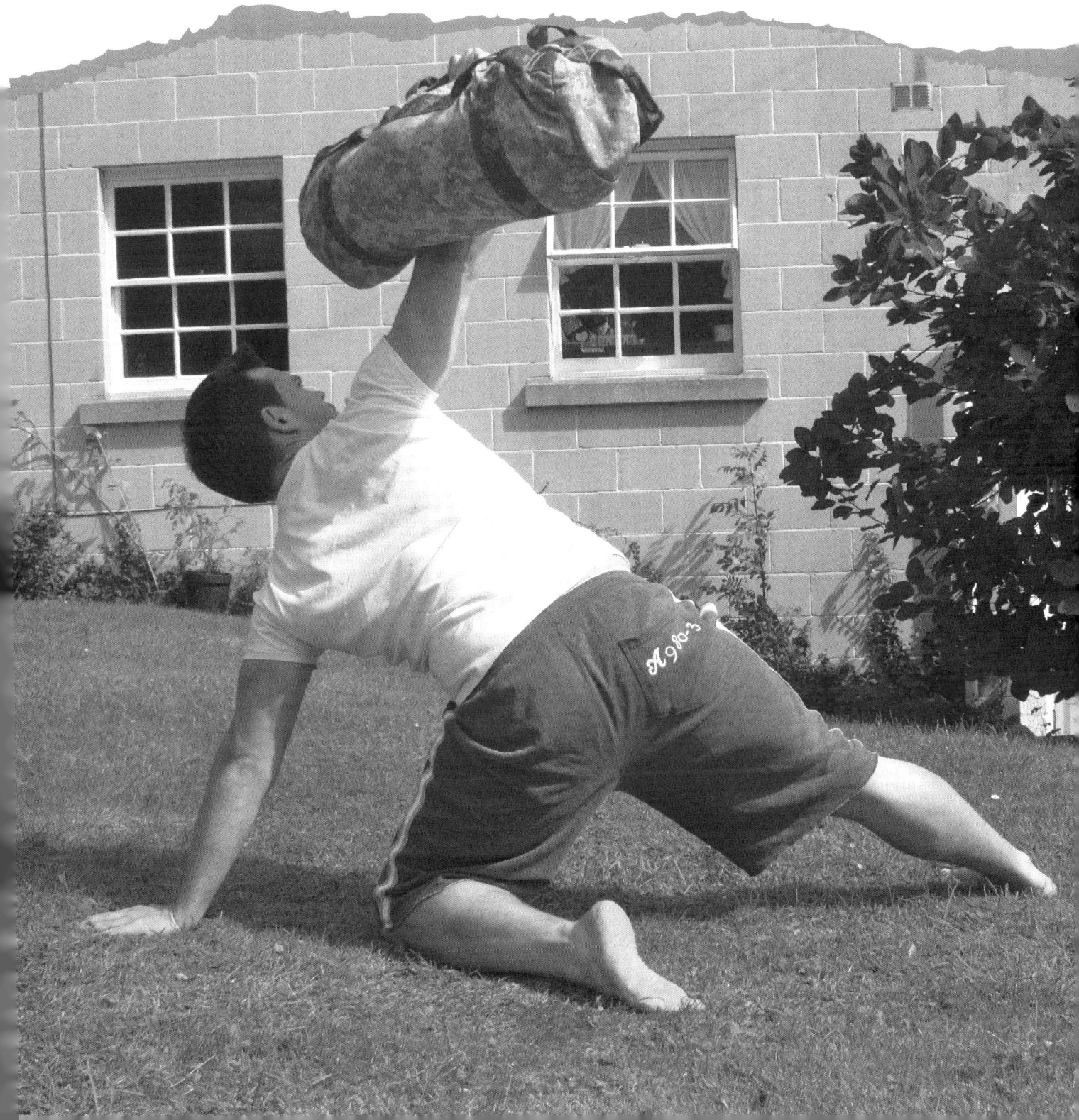

FULL BODY

Sandbag Thruster

The Thruster, or Squat and Press, is a great full-body exercise that will challenge everyone - even at moderate loads. Including both a lower body and an upper body exercise in one movement also qualifies it as an exercise that gives "a lot of bang for your buck". For those short on time it delivers outstanding results. It is essentially made up of the Sandbag Front Squat and the Sandbag Overhead Press.

Technique

- Start as you would for a Sandbag Front Squat
- As you begin to come out of the bottom of the squat, drive the sandbag upwards
- This extension of the arms should coincide with the hip and knee extension in the lower body - so that legs and arms straighten at the same time
- Return the sandbag to the Sandbag Front Squat position and repeat

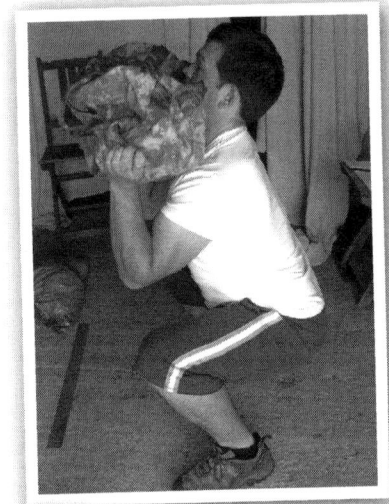

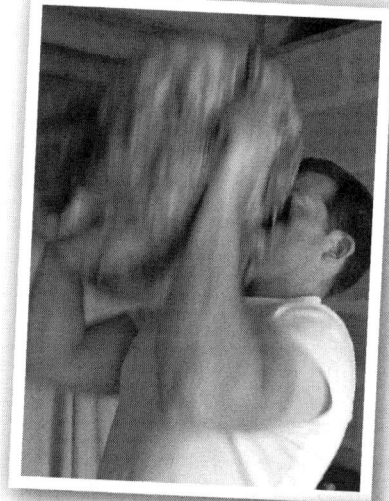

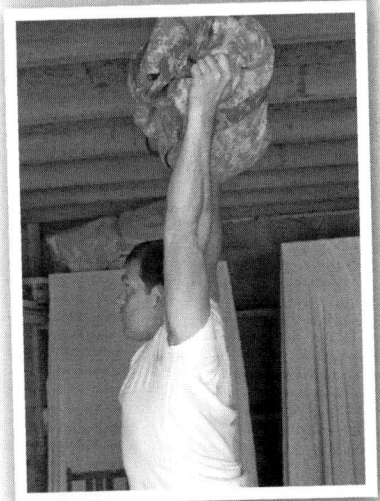

Sandbag Load Carry

The Sandbag Load Carry is exactly what it says - a way to transport the sandbag over a set distance. Carrying heavy objects is a great way to build strength and conditioning and the sandbag is no exception. There are a variety of different ways in which you can hold the sandbag (pictured below).

Technique

- Get the sandbag into your desired position
- Walk or run the required distance
- Ensure that you brace your core muscles to provide support as you move

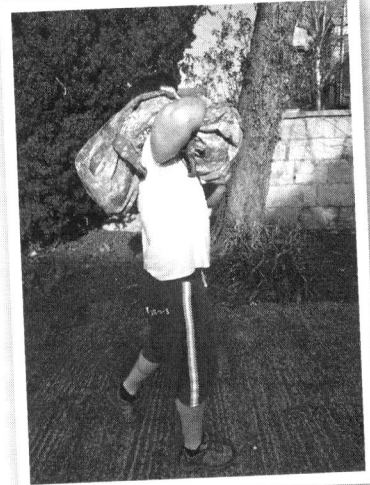

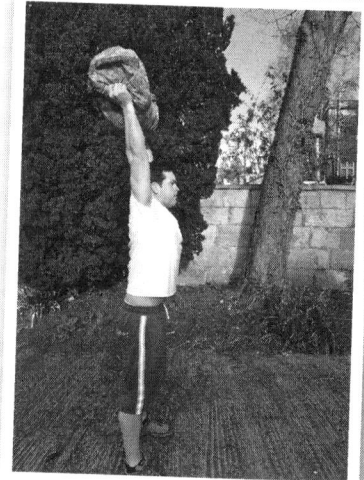

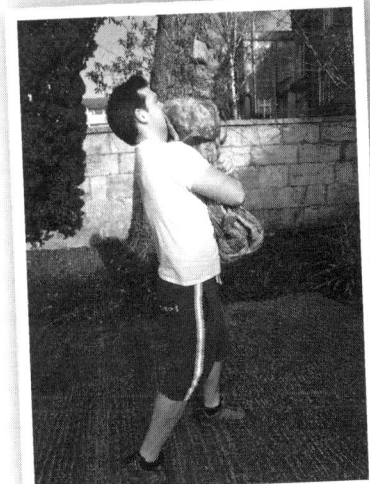

Sandbag Single Arm Swing

The Sandbag Single Arm Swing develops strength and power in the posterior chain muscles. Traditionally a kettlebell exercise, the sandbag variation requires more control.

Technique

- Take hold of a sandbag
- Set yourself with your chest high and hips backwards
- Keep the core braced and start to swing the sandbag up towards chest/head height - take a few swings to get here if you need to
- The power should come from your hips (backwards and forwards)
- Keep the spine in neutral

Variations

- Try a swing with 2 hands

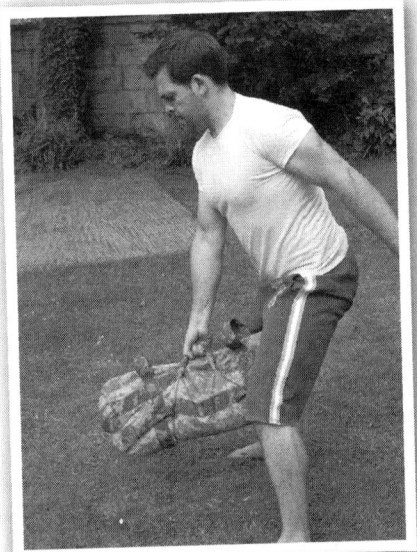

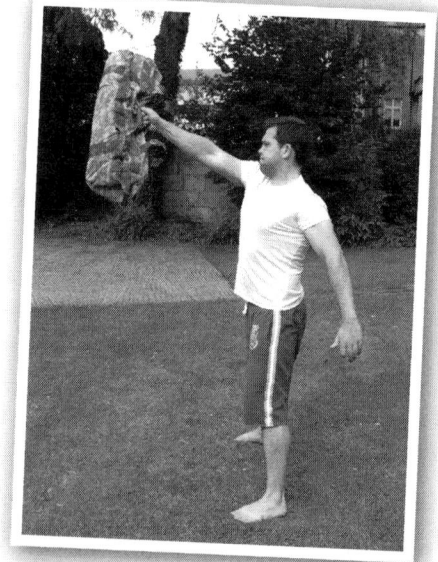

Sandbag Get Up

The Sandbag Get Up is another exercise that is traditionally done with either a kettlebell or a dumbbell. Using an unstable object like the sandbag makes for a much more challenging movement.

Technique

- Take hold of the sandbag in either one hand or across one shoulder
- Powerfully roll out onto your elbow on the opposite side
- Keep a wide base with your legs when you do this
- Push up onto your opposite hand
- Get your legs under you - ideally in a lunge position
- Stand up fully
- Return to the ground and repeat

Variations

- Perform the movement with the sandbag across the shoulder or in your extended arm

Sandbag Get Up

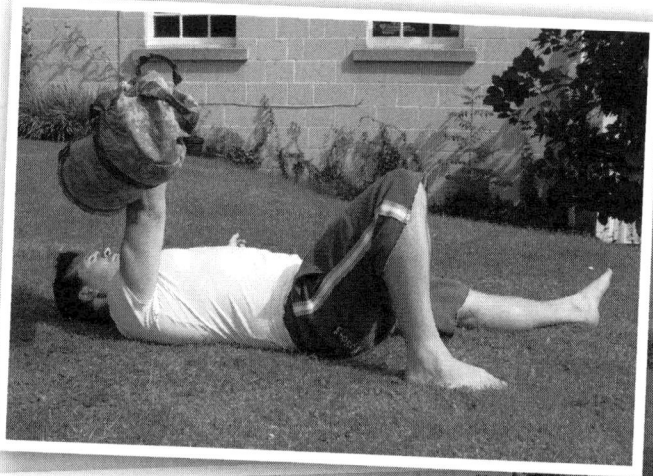

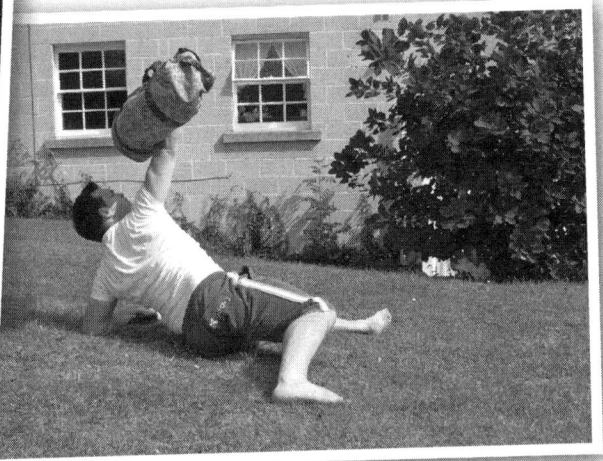

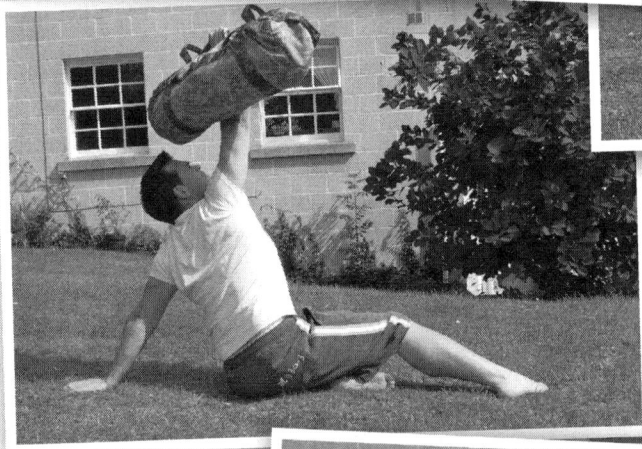

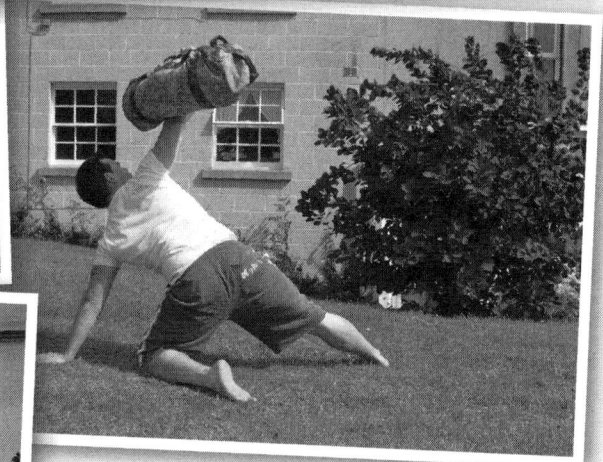

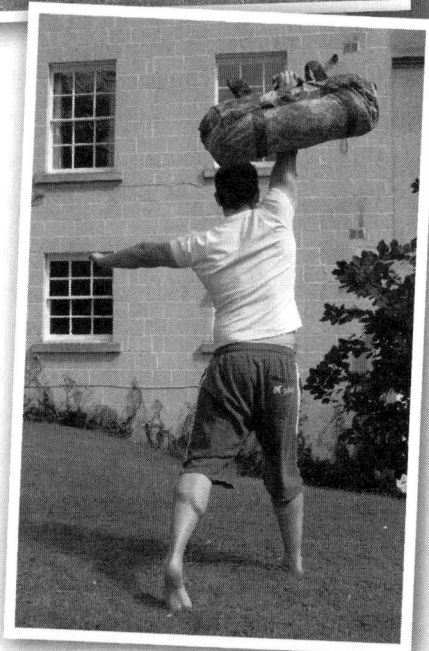

Sandbag Shoulder Get Up

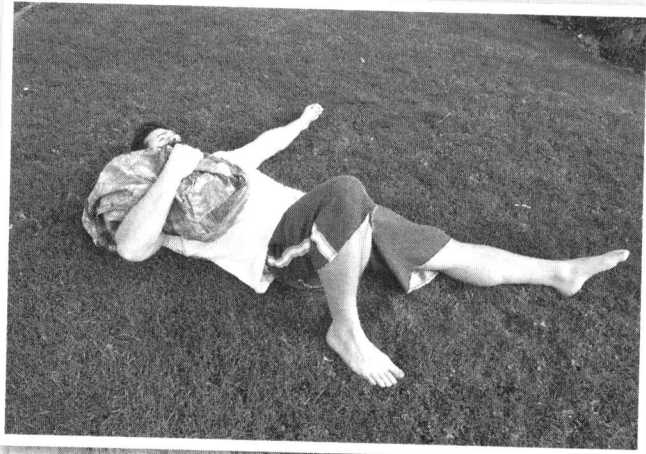

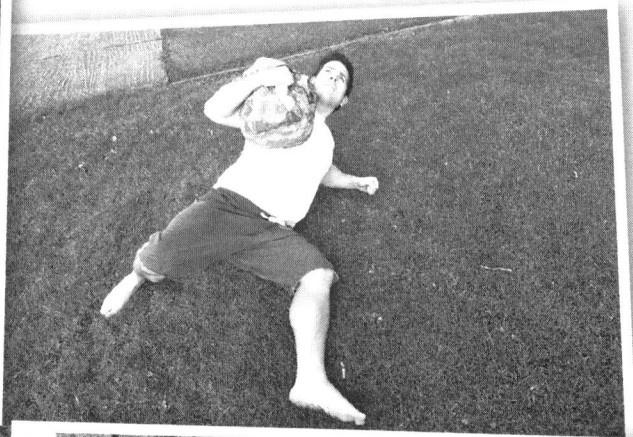

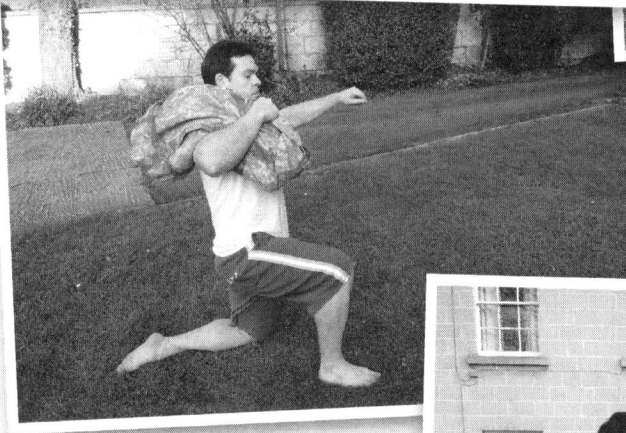

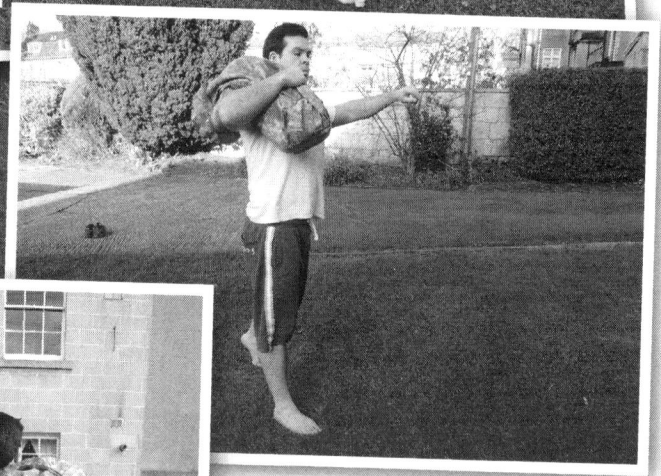

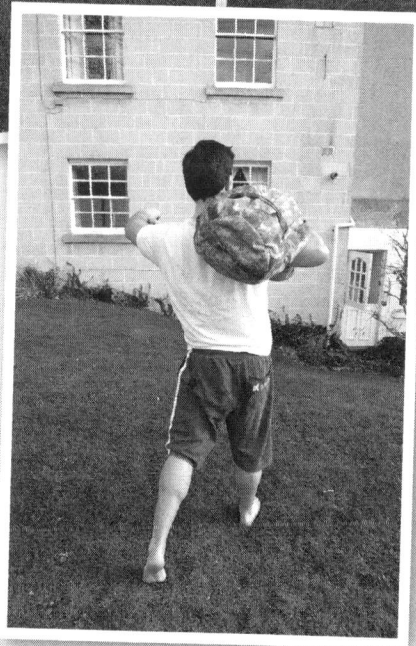

Burpee

The Burpee is a tough, full body agility and conditioning movement. Universally hated by most people (this normally puts an exercise in the 'important' category), the Burpee can be done anywhere.

Technique

- Start the exercise by bending down and placing your hands on the ground
- Shoot your legs out behind you, into a press/push up position
- Perform a full press/push up and then launch yourself back up onto your feet
- Stand up and perform a big upwards jump, reaching up as high as possible with your hands

Variations

- The Burpee can be performed without the Press/Push Up or with a modified Press/Push Up (knees on the ground)
- Try a lateral jump (sideways jump) over an object rather than an upwards jump
- Try a Box Jump rather than an upwards jump

Burpee

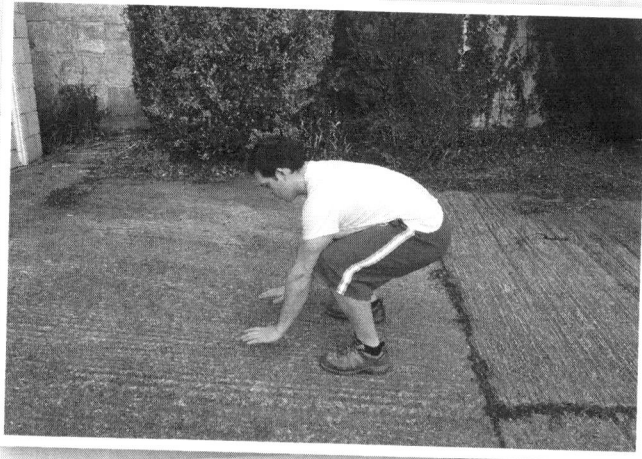
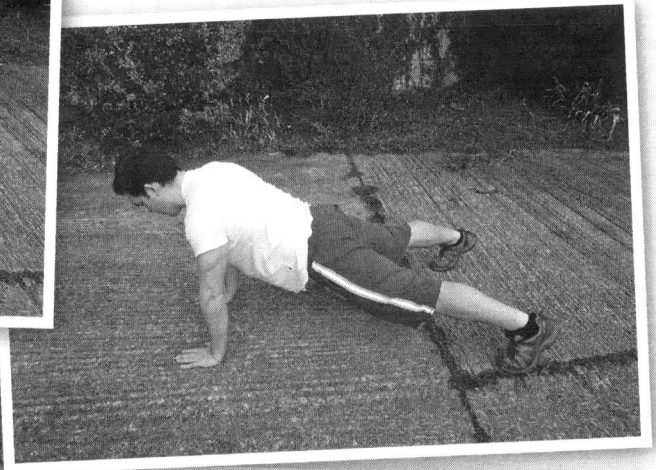
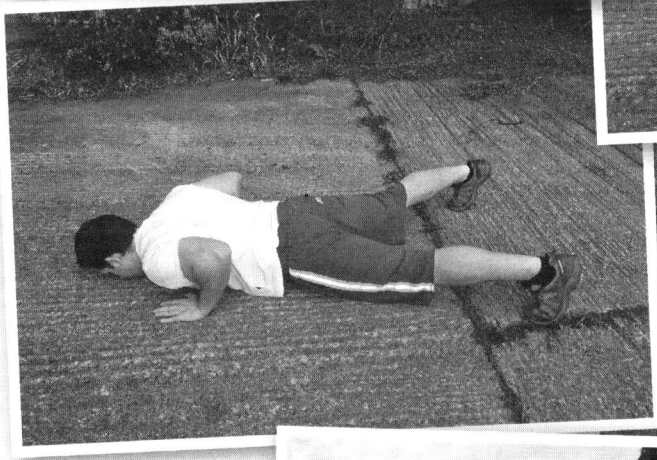
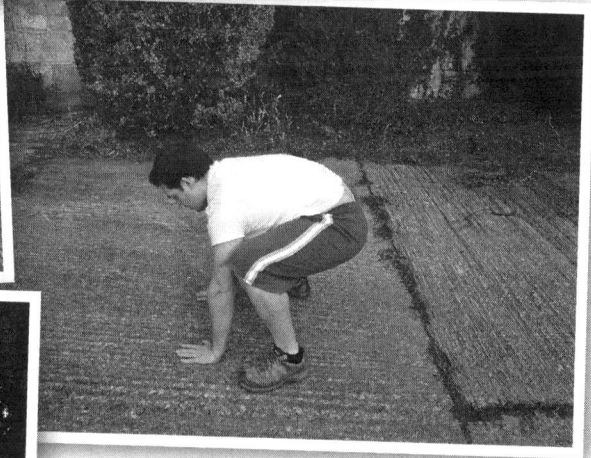
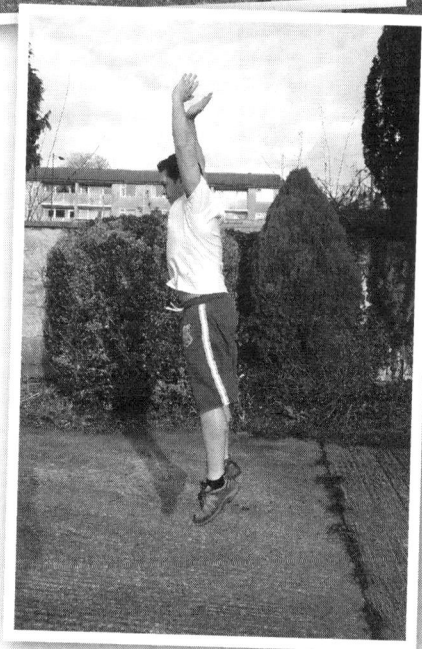

Skipping

Skipping is great for agility, coordination and general conditioning. Infinite progressions mean that you can get a lot from this simple exercise.

Technique

- Stay light on your feet throughout
- Keep the head up high
- Try to maintain a natural rhythm

Variations

- Double-Unders are done by performing a double rotation of the rope between each jump
- Experiment with different landings

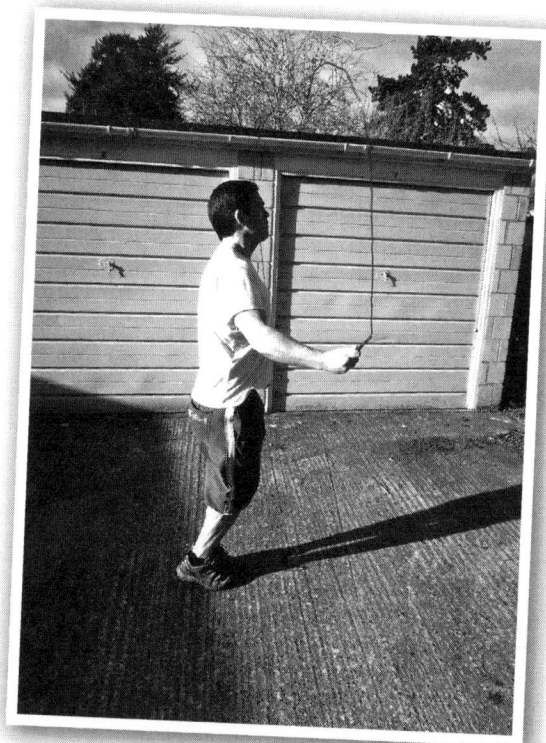

FULL BODY

Programmes

I have included 3 programmes: Beginner, Intermediate and Advanced. Each week contains 4 sessions - 2 strength sessions and 2 high intensity metabolic conditioning sessions. If you can't manage 4 sessions per week then do what you can, following the sessions in the order they are listed. If you are not familiar with following a programme of this type please read the notes first - they will explain, in detail, how you should follow this programme.

You will notice that the sessions are repeated during the course of the programme - this is your opportunity to chart progress against previous performance. So, be sure to record how well you do each session. There is also a Sandbag Challenge session at the beginning and end of each programme - this is another opportunity for you to test your progress.

If you are not used to working out with sandbags then take the time to learn the exercises and determine the correct weight for your sandbag before performing any of the sessions at high intensity. There is also a rough sandbag weight guide for men and women in the FAQ of this guide.

Sandbag Fitness is designed to be followed in conjunction with additional activity such as running, swimming or any other sport.

Programme Notes

Strength Sessions

- Take as much rest as you need between sets - you need to encourage high quality work and lift as much weight as possible

- If you are able to complete more repetitions or sets than the recommended then you need to increase the weight of your sandbag

- Over time you should aim to improve the amount of weight you can lift in your sandbag

- What is "5X5"?
  This refers to the number of repetitions and sets (reps X sets). Unless specified, you should complete 5 repetitions of the exercise, then rest as much as you need to. Repeat this for the given number of sets - in this case a total of 5. You would then move onto the next exercise.

- What is a "set to failure"?
  This refers to completing as many repetitions of an exercise, with good technique, as you can. If multiple sets are required, rest as needed (or as recommended) before repeating.

Programme Notes

Conditioning Sessions

- Unless specified you are trying to work as hard and as fast as possible, while still maintaining good technique

- Unless specified you should have a "running clock" for all of your conditioning sessions - this will include any time that you need to rest

- Over time you should try to improve times and scores for all of your workouts

- What is a "round"?
  A "round" refers to a series of exercises completed in sequence with no rest in between.

BEGINNERS PROGRAMME

"The beginning is the most important part of the work."

Plato

Week 1: Sandbag Challenge!

Do the exercises in the order that they are listed and record your performance. Aim to work as hard as you can and get the best possible score.

Take 5 minutes rest between each exercise.

- Press/Push Up - perform as many repetitions as possible
- Air Squat - perform as many repetitions as possible
- Plank - hold the position for as long as possible

- Sandbag Overhead Press - take a moderately heavy sandbag as perform as many repetitions as possible
- Sandbag Back Squat - take a moderately heavy sandbag and perform as many repetitions as possible

- Run 1km - run as fast as possible

Take the rest of this week off to recover and prepare for the start of the programme

Week 2: Strength

Strength Session 1:

Sandbag Deadlift: 5X5
Sandbag Back Squat: 5X5
Pull Ups: 3 sets to failure
Round-the-Worlds: 3 sets of 10-20 repetitions in each direction

Strength Session 2:

Sandbag Front Squat: 5X5
Sandbag Clean: 5X5
Sandbag Overhead Press: 5X5

Week 2: Strength

Workout	Exercise	Reps/Weight	Reps/Weight	Reps/Weight	Reps/Weight	Reps/Weight
Strength session 1	Sandbag Deadlift	/	/	/	/	/
	Sandbag Back Squat	/	/	/	/	/
	Pull Ups					
	Round-the-Worlds	/	/	/		
Strength session 2	Sandbag Front Squat	/	/	/	/	/
	Sandbag Clean	/	/	/	/	/
	Sandbag Overhead Press	/	/	/	/	/

Week 2: Conditioning

Conditioning Session 1:

800m run. 30 Sandbag Clean. 800m run.

Conditioning Session 2:

25 Box Jumps, 25 Sandbag High Pulls, 25 Sandbag Push Press. 3 rounds.

Workout	Exercise	Weight	Time
Conditioning session 1	800m run. 30 Sandbag Clean. 800m run.		
Conditioning session 2	25 Box Jumps, 25 Sandbag High Pulls, 25 Sandbag Push Press. 3 rounds.		

Week 3: Strength

Strength Session 1:

Sandbag Deadlift: 5X5
Sandbag Thruster: 5X5
Pull Ups: 3 sets to failure
Round-the-Worlds: 3 sets of 10-20 repetitions in each direction

Strength Session 2:

Sandbag Back Squat: 5X5
Sandbag Push Press: 5X5
Knees-to-Elbows: 3 sets to failure

Week 3: Strength

Workout	Exercise	Reps/Weight	Reps/Weight	Reps/Weight	Reps/Weight	Reps/Weight
Strength session 1	Sandbag Deadlift	/	/	/	/	/
	Sandbag Thruster	/	/	/	/	/
	Pull Ups					
	Round-the-Worlds	/	/	/		
Strength session 2	Sandbag Back Squat	/	/	/	/	/
	Sandbag Push Press	/	/	/	/	/
	Knees-to-Elbows					

Week 3: Conditioning

Conditioning Session 1:

10 Knees-to-Elbows, 15 Sandbag Zercher Squats, 20 Sandbag Overhead Press. 5 rounds. 30 seconds rest between rounds.

Conditioning Session 2:

400m run. 10 Sandbag Back Squats, 20 Box Jumps. 5 Rounds. 400m run.

Workout	Exercise	Weight	Time
Conditioning session 1	10 Knees-to-Elbows, 15 Sandbag Zercher Squats, 20 Sandbag Overhead Press. 5 rounds. 30 seconds rest between rounds.		
Conditioning session 2	400m run. 10 Sandbag Back Squats, 20 Box Jumps. 5 Rounds. 400m run.		

Week 4: Strength

Strength Session 1:

Sandbag Deadlift: 5X5
Sandbag Back Squat: 5X5
Pull Ups: 3 sets to failure
Round-the-Worlds: 3 sets of 10-20 repetitions

Strength Session 2:

Sandbag Front Squat: 5X5
Sandbag Clean: 5X5
Sandbag Overhead Press: 5X5

Week 4: Strength

Workout	Exercise	Reps/Weight	Reps/Weight	Reps/Weight	Reps/Weight	Reps/Weight
Strength session 1	Sandbag Deadlift	/	/	/	/	/
	Sandbag Back Squat	/	/	/	/	/
	Pull Ups					
	Round-the-Worlds	/	/	/		
Strength session 2	Sandbag Front Squat	/	/	/	/	/
	Sandbag Clean	/	/	/	/	/
	Sandbag Overhead Press	/	/	/	/	/

Week 4: Conditioning

Conditioning Session 1:

5 Pull Ups, 10 Sandbag Deadlifts, 10 Press Ups. 10 rounds.

Conditioning Session 2:

10 Air Squats, 10 Sandbag High Pulls, 10 Sandbag Push Press, 10 Sit Ups. As many rounds as possible in 15 minutes.

Workout	Exercise	Weight	Time
Conditioning session 1	5 Pull Ups, 10 Sandbag Deadlifts, 10 Press Ups. 10 rounds.		
Conditioning session 2	10 Air Squats, 10 Sandbag High Pulls, 10 Sandbag Push Jerks, 10 Sit Ups. As many rounds as possible in 15 minutes		Rounds x

Week 5: Strength

Strength Session 1:

Sandbag Deadlift: 5X5
Sandbag Thruster: 5X5
Pull Ups: 3 sets to failure
Round-the-Worlds: 3 sets of 10-20 repetitions in each direction

Strength Session 2:

Sandbag Back Squat: 5X5
Sandbag Clean and Push Jerk: 5X5
Knees-to-Elbows: 3 sets to failure

Week 5: Strength

Workout	Exercise	Reps/Weight	Reps/Weight	Reps/Weight	Reps/Weight	Reps/Weight
Strength session 1	Sandbag Deadlift	/	/	/	/	/
	Sandbag Thruster	/	/	/	/	/
	Pull Ups					
	Round-the-Worlds	/	/	/		
Strength session 2	Sandbag Back Squat	/	/	/	/	/
	Sandbag Clean and Push Jerk	/	/	/	/	/
	Knees-to-Elbows					

Week 5: Conditioning

Conditioning Session 1:

10 Sandbag Push Press,10 Sit Ups,10 Sandbag Back Squats,10 Pull Ups. As many rounds as possible in 20 minutes.

Conditioning Session 2:

15-1 of Press/Push Ups, Box Jumps and Sandbag Zercher Squats. Complete 15 repetitions of each exercise, then 14 etc.

Workout	Exercise	Weight	Time
Conditioning session 1	10 Sandbag Push Press,10 Sit Ups,10 Sandbag Back Squats,10 Pull Ups. As many rounds as possible in 20 minutes.		Rounds x
Conditioning session 2	15-1 of Press/Push Ups, Box Jumps and Sandbag Zercher Squats. Complete 15 repetitions of each exercise, then 14 etc.		

Week 6: Strength

Strength Session 1:

Sandbag Deadlift: 5X5
Sandbag Back Squat: 5X5
Pull Ups: 4 sets to failure
Round-the-Worlds: 3 sets of 10-20 repetitions

Strength Session 2:

Sandbag Front Squat: 5X5
Sandbag Clean: 5X5
Sandbag Overhead Press: 5X5

Week 6: Strength

Workout	Exercise	Reps/ Weight	Reps/ Weight	Reps/ Weight	Reps/ Weight	Reps/ Weight
Strength session 1	Sandbag Deadlift	/	/	/	/	/
	Sandbag Back Squat	/	/	/	/	/
	Pull Ups					
	Round-the-Worlds	/	/	/		
Strength session 2	Sandbag Front Squat	/	/	/	/	/
	Sandbag Clean	/	/	/	/	/
	Sandbag Overhead Press	/	/	/	/	/

Week 6: Conditioning

Conditioning Session 1:

800m run. 50 Sandbag Clean and Press. 800m run.

Conditioning Session 2:

25 Box Jumps, 25 Sandbag High Pulls, 25 Sandbag Push Press. 3 rounds.

Workout	Exercise	Weight	Time
Conditioning session 1	800m run. 50 Sandbag Clean & Press. 800m run.		
Conditioning session 2	25 Box Jumps, 25 Sandbag High Pulls, 25 Sandbag Push Press. 3 rounds.		

Week 7: Strength

Strength Session 1:

Sandbag Deadlift: 5X5
Sandbag Thruster: 5X5
Pull Ups: 4 sets to failure
Round-the-Worlds: 3 sets of 10-20 repetitions in each direction

Strength Session 2:

Sandbag Back Squat: 5X5
Sandbag Push Jerk: 5X5
Knees-to-Elbows: 4 sets to failure

Week 7: Strength

Workout	Exercise	Reps/Weight	Reps/Weight	Reps/Weight	Reps/Weight	Reps/Weight
Strength session 1	Sandbag Deadlift	/	/	/	/	/
	Sandbag Thruster	/	/	/	/	/
	Pull Ups					
	Round-the-Worlds	/	/	/		
Strength session 2	Sandbag Back Squat	/	/	/	/	/
	Sandbag Clean and Push Jerk	/	/	/	/	/
	Knees-to-Elbows					

Week 7: Conditioning

Conditioning Session 1:

10 Knees-to-Elbows, 15 Sandbag Zercher Squats, 20 Sandbag Overhead Press. 5 rounds. 30 seconds rest between rounds.

Conditioning Session 2:

400m run. 10 Sandbag Back Squats, 20 Box Jumps. 5 Rounds. 400m run.

Workout	Exercise	Weight	Time
Conditioning session 1	10 Knees-to-Elbows, 15 Sandbag Zercher Squats, 20 Sandbag Overhead Press. 5 rounds. 30 seconds rest between rounds.		
Conditioning session 2	400m run. 10 Sandbag Back Squats, 20 Box Jumps. 5 Rounds. 400m run.		

Week 8: Strength

Strength Session 1:

Sandbag Deadlift: 5X5
Sandbag Back Squat: 5X5
Pull Ups: 5 sets to failure
Round-the-Worlds: 3 sets of 10-20 repetitions in each direction

Strength Session 2:

Sandbag Front Squat: 5X5
Sandbag Clean: 5X5
Sandbag Overhead Press: 5X5

Week 8: Strength

Workout	Exercise	Reps/ Weight	Reps/ Weight	Reps/ Weight	Reps/ Weight	Reps/ Weight
Strength session 1	Sandbag Deadlift	/	/	/	/	/
	Sandbag Back Squat	/	/	/	/	/
	Pull Ups					
	Round-the-Worlds	/	/	/		
Strength session 2	Sandbag Front Squat	/	/	/	/	/
	Sandbag Clean	/	/	/	/	/
	Sandbag Overhead Press	/	/	/	/	/

Week 8: Conditioning

Conditioning Session 1:

5 Pull Ups, 10 Sandbag Deadlifts, 10 Press Ups. 10 rounds.

Conditioning Session 2:

10 Air Squats, 10 Sandbag High Pulls, 10 Sandbag Overhead Press, 10 Sit Ups. As many rounds as possible in 15 minutes.

Workout	Exercise	Weight	Time
Conditioning session 1	5 Pull Ups, 10 Sandbag Deadlifts, 10 Press Ups. 10 rounds.		
Conditioning session 2	10 Air Squats, 10 Sandbag High Pulls, 10 Sandbag Overhead Press, 10 Sit Ups. As many rounds as possible in 15 minutes.		Rounds x

Week 9: Strength

Strength Session 1:

Sandbag Deadlift: 5X5
Sandbag Thruster: 5X5
Pull Ups: 5 sets to failure
Round-the-Worlds: 3 sets of 10-20 repetitions in each direction

Strength Session 2:

Sandbag Back Squat: 5X5
Sandbag Clean and Push Jerk: 5X5
Knees-to-Elbows: 5 sets to failure

Week 9: Strength

Workout	Exercise	Reps/Weight	Reps/Weight	Reps/Weight	Reps/Weight	Reps/Weight
Strength session 1	Sandbag Deadlift	/	/	/	/	/
	Sandbag Thruster	/	/	/	/	/
	Pull Ups					
	Round-the-Worlds	/	/	/		
Strength session 2	Sandbag Back Squat	/	/	/	/	/
	Sandbag Clean and Push Jerk	/	/	/	/	/
	Knees-to-Elbows					

Week 9: Conditioning

Conditioning Session 1:

10 Sandbag Push Press,10 Sit Ups,10 Sandbag Back Squats,10 Pull Ups. As many rounds as possible in 20 minutes.

Conditioning Session 2:

15-1 of Press/Push Ups, Box Jumps and Sandbag Zercher Squats. Complete 15 repetitions of each exercise, then 14 etc.

Workout	Exercise	Weight	Time
Conditioning session 1	10 Sandbag Push Press,10 Sit Ups,10 Sandbag Back Squats,10 Pull Ups. As many rounds as possible in 20 minutes.		Rounds x
Conditioning session 2	15-1 of Press/Push Ups, Box Jumps and Sandbag Zercher Squats. Complete 15 repetitions of each exercise, then 14 etc.		

Week 10: Sandbag Challenge!

Do the exercises in the order that they are listed and record your performance. Aim to work as hard as you can and get the best possible score. You should aim to beat your previous best scores for the exercises below.

Take 5 minutes rest between each exercise.

- Press/Push Up - perform as many repetitions as possible
- Air Squat - perform as many repetitions as possible
- Plank - hold the position for as long as possible

- Sandbag Overhead Press - take a moderately heavy sandbag as perform as many repetitions as possible. Use the same weight sandbag as in Week 1
- Sandbag Back Squat - take a moderately heavy sandbag and perform as many repetitions as possible. Use the same weight sandbag as in Week 1

- Run 1km - run as fast as possible

Did you improve over the past 10 weeks?

Take the rest of this week off to recover and prepare for the start of the next programme

CONGRATULATIONS!

You're through the Beginners Programme!

INTERMEDIATE PROGRAMME

"It's easy to have faith in yourself and have discipline when you're a winner, when you're number one. What you got to have is faith and discipline when you're not a winner."

Vince Lombardi

Week 1: Sandbag Challenge!

Do the exercises in the order that they are listed and record your performance. Aim to work as hard as you can and get the best possible score.

Take 5 minutes rest between each exercise.

- **Press/Push Up** - perform as many repetitions as possible
- **Knees-to-Elbows** - perform as many repetitions as possible
- **Pull Ups** - perform as many repetitions as possible

- **Sandbag Thruster** - take a moderately heavy sandbag as perform as many repetitions as possible
- **Sandbag Deadlift** - take a heavy sandbag and perform as many repetitions as possible
- **Sandbag Windmill** - perform as many repetitions as possible. Repeat with both arms
- **Sandbag Zercher Squat** - take a moderately heavy sandbag and perform as many repetitions as possible

- **Run 2km** - run as fast as possible

Take the rest of this week off to recover and prepare for the start of the programme

Week 2: Strength

Strength Session 1:

Sandbag Suitcase Deadlift: 5X5
Sandbag Zercher Squat: 5X5
Sandbag Floor Press: 5X5
Sandbag Windmill: 3X5
Lower Back Raise: 3 sets to failure

Strength Session 2:

Sandbag Deadlift: 5X5
Sandbag Back Squat: 5X5
Sandbag Overhead Press: 5X5
Pull Ups: 4 sets to failure
Plank: 3 sets to failure

Week 2: Strength

Workout	Exercise	Reps/Weight	Reps/Weight	Reps/Weight	Reps/Weight	Reps/Weight
Strength session 1	Sandbag Suitcase Deadlift	/	/	/	/	/
	Sandbag Zercher Squat	/	/	/	/	/
	Sandbag Floor Press	/	/	/	/	/
	Sandbag Windmill	/	/	/		
	Lower Back Raise					
Strength session 2	Sandbag Deadlift	/	/	/	/	/
	Sandbag Back Squat	/	/	/	/	/
	Sandbag Overhead Press	/	/	/	/	/
	Pull Ups					
	Plank					

Week 2: Conditioning

Conditioning Session 1:

Sandbag Hill Sprint (sprint up a 40-60m hill carrying a sandbag). 10 Sandbag Back Squats at the top of the hill. As many rounds as possible in 20 minutes.

Conditioning Session 2:

15-1 of Sandbag Shouldering, Sit-Ups and Press/Push Ups. Complete 15 repetitions of each exercise, then 14 etc.

Workout	Exercise	Weight	Time
Conditioning session 1	Sandbag Hill Sprint (sprint up a 40-60m hill carrying a sandbag). 10 Sandbag Back Squats at the top of the hill. As many rounds as possible in 20 minutes.		
Conditioning session 2	15-1 of Sandbag Shouldering, Sit-Ups and Press/Push Ups. Complete 15 repetitions of each exercise, then 14 etc.		

Week 3: Strength

Strength Session 1:

Sandbag Clean: 5X5
Sandbag Bear Hug Squat: 5X5
Sandbag Bent Over Row: 5X5
Sandbag Bent Press: 5X5
Lower Back Raise: 3 sets to failure

Strength Session 2:

Sandbag Deadlift: 5X5
Sandbag Back Squat: 5X5
Sandbag Push Jerk: 3X5
Sandbag Shouldering: 3X10
Plank: 3 sets to failure

Week 3: Strength

Workout	Exercise	Reps/Weight	Reps/Weight	Reps/Weight	Reps/Weight	Reps/Weight
Strength session 1	Sandbag Clean	/	/	/	/	/
	Sandbag Bear Hug Squat	/	/	/	/	/
	Sandbag Bent Over Row	/	/	/	/	/
	Sandbag Bent Press	/	/	/		
	Lower Back Raise					
Strength session 2	Sandbag Deadlift	/	/	/	/	/
	Sandbag Back Squat	/	/	/	/	/
	Sandbag Push Jerk	/	/	/		
	Sandbag Shouldering	/	/	/		
	Plank					

Week 3: Conditioning

Conditioning Session 1:

800 m run. 50 Sandbag Cleans, 50 Sandbag Push Press, 50 Sandbag Deadlifts. 800m run.

Conditioning Session 2:

100 Sandbag Push Press, 100 Sandbag Zercher Squats, 100 Sandbag Deadlifts, 100 Sandbag Cleans. Complete in any order.

Workout	Exercise	Weight	Time
Conditioning session 1	800 m run. 50 Sandbag Cleans, 50 Sandbag Push Press, 50 Sandbag Deadlifts. 800m run.		
Conditioning session 2	100 Sandbag Push Press, 100 Sandbag Zercher Squats, 100 Sandbag Deadlifts, 100 Sandbag Cleans. Complete in any order.		

Week 4: Strength

Strength Session 1:

Sandbag Front Squat: 5X5
Sandbag Snatch: 3X5
Sandbag Push Press: 5X5
Sandbag Get Up: 3X5
Lower Back Raise: 3 sets to failure

Strength Session 2:

Sandbag Deadlift: 5X5
Sandbag Back Squat: 5X5
Handstand Press/Push Ups: 3 sets to failure
Gorilla Pull Ups: 3 sets to failure
Plank: 3 sets to failure

Week 4: Strength

Workout	Exercise	Reps/Weight	Reps/Weight	Reps/Weight	Reps/Weight	Reps/Weight
Strength session 1	Sandbag Front Squat	/	/	/	/	/
	Sandbag Snatch	/	/	/		
	Sandbag Push Press	/	/	/	/	/
	Sandbag Get Up	/	/	/		
	Lower Back Raise					
Strength session 2	Sandbag Deadlift	/	/	/	/	/
	Sandbag Back Squat	/	/	/	/	/
	Handstand Press/ Push Ups					
	Gorilla Pull Ups					
	Plank					

Week 4: Conditioning

Conditioning Session 1:

100m Load Carry, 10 Burpees, 10 Box Jumps. 10 rounds.

Conditioning Session 2:

100 Sandbag Overhead Press. There is a 100 Skip penalty for every break you take during the set.

Workout	Exercise	Weight	Time
Conditioning session 1	100m Load Carry, 10 Burpees, 10 Box Jumps. 10 rounds.		
Conditioning session 2	100 Sandbag Overhead Press. There is a 100 Skip penalty for every break you take during the set.		Rounds x

Week 5: Strength

Strength Session 1:

Sandbag Thruster: 5X5
Sandbag Walking Lunge: 3X10
Sandbag Shouldering: 3X10
Sandbag Good Morning: 3X10
Lower Back Raise: 3 sets to failure

Strength Session 2:

Sandbag Deadlift: 5X5
Sandbag Back Squat: 5X5
Sandbag Shoulder-to-Shoulder Press: 3X10
Hanging Leg Raises: 3 sets to failure
Plank: 3 sets to failure

Week 5: Strength

Workout	Exercise	Reps/ Weight	Reps/ Weight	Reps/ Weight	Reps/ Weight	Reps/ Weight
Strength session 1	Sandbag Thruster	/	/	/	/	/
	Sandbag Walking Lunge	/	/	/		
	Sandbag Shouldering	/	/	/		
	Sandbag Good Morning	/	/	/		
	Lower Back Raise					
Strength session 2	Sandbag Deadlift	/	/	/	/	/
	Sandbag Back Squat	/	/	/	/	/
	Sandbag Shoulder-to Shoulder	/	/	/		
	Hanging Leg Raises					
	Plank					

Week 5: Conditioning

Conditioning Session 1:

100m Hill Sprint (unloaded), 10 Sandbag Thrusters. As many rounds as possible in 15 minutes.

Conditioning Session 2:

20 Sandbag Walking Lunges, 20 Sandbag Shouldering, 20 Sandbag Bent Over Row, 20 T Press/Push Ups, 20 Sandbag Single Arm Swings. 3 rounds.

Workout	Exercise	Weight	Time
Conditioning session 1	100m Hill Sprint (unloaded), 10 Sandbag Thrusters. As many rounds as possible in 15 minutes.		Rounds x
Conditioning session 2	20 Sandbag Walking Lunges, 20 Sandbag Shouldering, 20 Sandbag Bent Over Row, 20 T Press/ Push Ups, 20 Sandbag Single Arm Swings. 3 rounds.		

Week 6: Strength

Strength Session 1:

Sandbag Suitcase Deadlift: 5X5
Sandbag Zercher Squat: 5X5
Sandbag Floor Press: 5X5
Sandbag Windmill: 4X5
Lower Back Raise: 4 sets to failure

Strength Session 2:

Sandbag Deadlift: 5X5
Sandbag Back Squat: 5X5
Sandbag Overhead Press: 5X5
Pull Ups: 5 sets to failure
Plank: 4 sets to failure

Week 6: Strength

Workout	Exercise	Reps/ Weight	Reps/ Weight	Reps/ Weight	Reps/ Weight	Reps/ Weight
Strength session 1	Sandbag Suitcase Deadlift	/	/	/	/	/
	Sandbag Zercher Squat	/	/	/	/	/
	Sandbag Floor Press	/	/	/	/	/
	Sandbag Windmill	/	/	/	/	
	Lower Back Raise					
Strength session 2	Sandbag Deadlift	/	/	/	/	/
	Sandbag Back Squat	/	/	/	/	/
	Sandbag Overhead Press	/	/	/	/	/
	Pull Ups					
	Plank					

Week 6: Conditioning

Conditioning Session 1:

Sandbag Hill Sprint (sprint up a 40-60m hill carrying a sandbag). 10 Sandbag Back Squats at the top of the hill. As many rounds as possible in 20 minutes.

Conditioning Session 2:

15-1 of Sandbag Shouldering, Sit-Ups and Press/Push Ups. Complete 15 repetitions of each exercise, then 14 etc.

Workout	Exercise	Weight	Time
Conditioning session 1	Sandbag Hill Sprint (sprint up a 40-60m hill carrying a sandbag). 10 Sandbag Back Squats at the top of the hill. As many rounds as possible in 20 minutes.		
Conditioning session 2	15-1 of Sandbag Shouldering, Sit-Ups and Press/Push Ups. Complete 15 repetitions of each exercise, then 14 etc.		

Week 7: Strength

Strength Session 1:

Sandbag Clean: 5X5
Sandbag Bear Hug Squat: 5X5
Sandbag Bent Over Row: 5X5
Sandbag Bent Press: 5X5
Lower Back Raise: 4 sets to failure

Strength Session 2:

Sandbag Deadlift: 5X5
Sandbag Back Squat: 5X5
Sandbag Push Jerk: 4X5
Sandbag Shouldering: 4X10
Plank: 4 sets to failure

Week 7: Strength

Workout	Exercise	Reps/Weight	Reps/Weight	Reps/Weight	Reps/Weight	Reps/Weight
Strength session 1	Sandbag Clean	/	/	/	/	/
	Sandbag Bear Hug Squat	/	/	/	/	/
	Sandbag Bent Over Row	/	/	/	/	/
	Sandbag Bent Press	/	/	/	/	/
	Lower Back Raise					
Strength session 2	Sandbag Deadlift	/	/	/	/	/
	Sandbag Back Squat	/	/	/	/	/
	Sandbag Push Jerk	/	/	/	/	
	Sandbag Shouldering	/	/	/	/	
	Plank					

Week 7: Conditioning

Conditioning Session 1:

800 m run. 50 Sandbag Cleans, 50 Sandbag Push Press, 50 Sandbag Deadlifts. 800m run.

Conditioning Session 2:

100 Sandbag Push Press, 100 Sandbag Zercher Squats, 100 Sandbag Deadlifts, 100 Sandbag Cleans. Complete in any order.

Workout	Exercise	Weight	Time
Conditioning session 1	800 m run. 50 Sandbag Cleans, 50 Sandbag Push Press, 50 Sandbag Deadlifts. 800m run.		
Conditioning session 2	100 Sandbag Push Press, 100 Sandbag Zercher Squats, 100 Sandbag Deadlifts, 100 Sandbag Cleans. Complete in any order.		

Week 8: Strength

Strength Session 1:

Sandbag Front Squat: 5X5
Sandbag Snatch: 4X5
Sandbag Push Press: 5X5
Sandbag Get Up: 4X5
Lower Back Raise: 4 sets to failure

Strength Session 2:

Sandbag Deadlift: 5X5
Sandbag Back Squat: 5X5
Handstand Press/Push Ups: 4 sets to failure
Gorilla Pull Ups: 4 sets to failure
Plank: 4 sets to failure

Week 8: Strength

Workout	Exercise	Reps/ Weight	Reps/ Weight	Reps/ Weight	Reps/ Weight	Reps/ Weight
Strength session 1	Sandbag Front Squat	/	/	/	/	/
	Sandbag Snatch	/	/	/	/	
	Sandbag Push Press	/	/	/	/	/
	Sandbag Get Up	/	/	/	/	
	Lower Back Raise					
Strength session 2	Sandbag Deadlift	/	/	/	/	/
	Sandbag Back Squat	/	/	/	/	/
	Handstand Press/ Push Ups					
	Gorilla Pull Ups					
	Plank					

Week 8: Conditioning

Conditioning Session 1:

100m Load Carry, 10 Burpees, 10 Box Jumps. 10 rounds.

Conditioning Session 2:

100 Sandbag Overhead Press. There is a 100 Skip penalty for every break you take during the set.

Workout	Exercise	Weight	Time
Conditioning session 1	100m Load Carry, 10 Burpees, 10 Box Jumps. 10 rounds.		
Conditioning session 2	100 Sandbag Overhead Press. There is a 100 Skip penalty for every break you take during the set.		Rounds x

Week 9: Strength

Strength Session 1:

Sandbag Thruster: 5X5
Sandbag Walking Lunge: 4X10
Sandbag Shouldering: 5X10
Sandbag Good Morning: 5X10
Lower Back Raise: 5 sets to failure

Strength Session 2:

Sandbag Deadlift: 5X5
Sandbag Back Squat: 5X5
Sandbag Shoulder-to-Shoulder Press: 4X10
Hanging Leg Raises: 4 sets to failure
Plank: 5 sets to failure

Week 9: Strength

Workout	Exercise	Reps/ Weight	Reps/ Weight	Reps/ Weight	Reps/ Weight	Reps/ Weight
Strength session 1	Sandbag Thruster	/	/	/	/	/
	Sandbag Walking Lunge	/	/	/	/	
	Sandbag Shouldering	/	/	/	/	/
	Sandbag Good Morning	/	/	/	/	/
	Lower Back Raise					
Strength session 2	Sandbag Deadlift	/	/	/	/	/
	Sandbag Back Squat	/	/	/	/	/
	Sandbag Shoulder-to Shoulder	/	/	/	/	
	Hanging Leg Raises					
	Plank					

Week 9: Conditioning

Conditioning Session 1:

100m Hill Sprint (unloaded), 10 Sandbag Thrusters. As many rounds as possible in 15 minutes.

Conditioning Session 2:

20 Sandbag Walking Lunges, 20 Sandbag Shouldering, 20 Sandbag Bent Over Row, 20 T Press/Push Ups, 20 Sandbag Single Arm Swings. 3 rounds.

Workout	Exercise	Weight	Time
Conditioning session 1	100m Hill Sprint (unloaded), 10 Sandbag Thrusters. As many rounds as possible in 15 minutes.		Rounds x
Conditioning session 2	20 Sandbag Walking Lunges, 20 Sandbag Shouldering, 20 Sandbag Bent Over Row, 20 T Press/ Push Ups, 20 Sandbag Single Arm Swings. 3 rounds.		

Week 10: Sandbag Challenge!

Do the exercises in the order that they are listed and record your performance. Aim to work as hard as you can and get the best possible score. You should aim to beat your previous best scores for the exercises below.

Take 5 minutes rest between each exercise.

- Press/Push Up - perform as many repetitions as possible
- Knees-to-Elbows - perform as many repetitions as possible
- Pull Ups - perform as many repetitions as possible

- Sandbag Thruster - take a moderately heavy sandbag as perform as many repetitions as possible
- Sandbag Deadlift - take a heavy sandbag and perform as many repetitions as possible
- Sandbag Windmill - perform as many repetitions as possible. Repeat with both arms
- Sandbag Zercher Squat - take a moderately heavy sandbag and perform as many repetitions as possible

- Run 2km - run as fast as possible

Did you improve over the past 10 weeks?

Take the rest of this week off to recover and prepare for the start of the next programme

CONGRATULATIONS!

You're through the Intermediate Programme!

ADVANCED PROGRAMME

"I've missed more than 9000 shots in my career. I've lost almost 300 games. 26 times, I've been trusted to take the game winning shot and missed. I've failed over and over and over again in my life. And that is why I succeed."

Michael Jordan

Week 1: Sandbag Challenge!

Do the exercises in the order that they are listed and record your performance. Aim to work as hard as you can and get the best possible score.

Take 5 minutes rest between each exercise.

- T Press/Push Ups - perform as many repetitions as possible
- Toes-to-Bar - perform as many repetitions as possible
- L Pull Ups - perform as many repetitions as possible
- Handstand Press/Push Ups - perform as many repetitions as possible

- Sandbag Overhead Walking Lunge - take a moderately heavy sandbag as perform as many repetitions as possible
- Sandbag Clean and Push Jerk - take a moderately heavy sandbag and perform as many repetitions as possible
- Sandbag Bent Press - perform as many repetitions as possible. Repeat with both arms
- Sandbag Shoulder Squat - take a moderately heavy sandbag and perform as many repetitions as possible

- Run 4km - run as fast as possible

Take the rest of this week off to recover and prepare for the start of the programme

Week 2: Strength

Strength Session 1:

Sandbag Deadlift: 5X5
Sandbag Clean: 5X5
Sandbag Bent Over Row: 5X5
Sandbag Good Mornings: 3X10
Handstand Press/Push Ups: 4 sets to failure

Strength Session 2:

Sandbag Shoulder Squat: 5X5
Sandbag Floor Press: 5X5
Gorilla Pull Ups: 4 sets to failure
Sandbag Shoulder Get Ups: 3X5
Sandbag Round-the-Worlds: 4X20

Week 2: Strength

Workout	Exercise	Reps/Weight	Reps/Weight	Reps/Weight	Reps/Weight	Reps/Weight
Strength session 1	Sandbag Deadlift	/	/	/	/	/
	Sandbag Clean	/	/	/	/	/
	Sandbag Bent Over Row	/	/	/	/	/
	Sandbag Good Mornings	/	/	/		
	Handstand Press/ Push Ups					
Strength session 2	Sandbag Shoulder Squat	/	/	/	/	/
	Sandbag Floor Press	/	/	/	/	/
	Gorilla Pull Ups					
	Sandbag Shoulder Get Ups	/	/	/		
	Sandbag Round-the-Worlds	/	/	/	/	

Week 2: Conditioning

Conditioning Session 1:

Sandbag Hill Sprint (sprint up a 40-60m hill carrying a sandbag). 10 Sandbag Floor Press at the bottom of the hill. As many rounds as possible in 20 minutes.

Conditioning Session 2:

150 Skips, 20 Burpees, 15 High Pulls, 10 Sandbag Thrusters. 5 rounds.

Workout	Exercise	Weight	Time
Conditioning session 1	Sandbag Hill Sprint (sprint up a 40-60m hill carrying a sandbag). 10 Sandbag Floor Press at the bottom of the hill. As many rounds as possible in 20 minutes.		
Conditioning session 2	150 Skips, 20 Burpees, 15 High Pulls, 10 Sandbag Thrusters. 5 rounds.		

Week 3: Strength

Strength Session 1:

Sandbag Suitcase Deadlift: 5X5
Sandbag Snatch: 3X5
Sandbag Push Jerk: 5X5
T Press/Push Ups: 4 sets to failure
Toes-to-Bar: 4 sets to failure

Strength Session 2:

Sandbag Zercher Squats: 5X5
Sandbag Overhead Press: 5X5
Sandbag High Pulls: 5X5
Gorilla Pull Ups: 4 sets to failure
Sandbag Windmills: 4X5

Week 3: Strength

Workout	Exercise	Reps/Weight	Reps/Weight	Reps/Weight	Reps/Weight	Reps/Weight
Strength session 1	Sandbag Suitcase Deadlift	/	/	/	/	/
	Sandbag Snatch	/	/	/		
	Sandbag Push Jerk	/	/	/	/	/
	T Press/Push Up					
	Toes-to-Bar					
Strength session 2	Sandbag Zercher Squats	/	/	/	/	/
	Sandbag Overhead Press	/	/	/	/	/
	Sandbag High Pulls	/	/	/	/	
	Gorilla Pull Ups					
	Sandbag Windmills	/	/	/	/	

Week 3: Conditioning

Conditioning Session 1:

5 Gorilla Pull Ups, 10 Handstand Press/Push Ups,15 Sandbag Shoulder Squats.
10 rounds.

Conditioning Session 2:

5 Sandbag Cleans, 5 Sandbag Push Jerks, 5 Sandbag Zercher Squats, 5
Sandbag Good Mornings.

Workout	Exercise	Weight	Time
Conditioning session 1	5 Gorilla Pull Ups, 10 Handstand Press/Push Ups,15 Sandbag Shoulder Squats. 10 rounds.		
Conditioning session 2	5 Sandbag Cleans, 5 Sandbag Push Jerks, 5 Sandbag Zercher Squats, 5 Sandbag Good Mornings.		

Week 4: Strength

Strength Session 1:

Sandbag Deadlift: 5X5
Sandbag Power Cleans: 5X5
Sandbag Bent Over Row: 5X5
Sandbag Good Mornings: 3X5
Sandbag Round-the-Worlds: 3 sets to failure

Strength Session 2:

Sandbag Front Squat: 5X5
Sandbag Floor Press: 5X5
Sandbag High Pulls: 5X5
L Pull Ups: 3 sets to failure
Sandbag Get Ups: 3X5

Week 4: Strength

Workout	Exercise	Reps/Weight	Reps/Weight	Reps/Weight	Reps/Weight	Reps/Weight
Strength session 1	Sandbag Deadlift	/	/	/	/	/
	Sandbag Power Cleans	/	/	/	/	/
	Sandbag Bent Over Row	/	/	/	/	/
	Sandbag Good Mornings	/	/	/		
	Sandbag Round-the-Worlds	/	/	/		
Strength session 2	Sandbag Front Squat	/	/	/	/	/
	Sandbag Floor Press	/	/	/	/	/
	Sandbag High Pulls	/	/	/	/	/
	L Pull Ups					
	Sandbag Get Ups	/	/	/		

Week 4: Conditioning

Conditioning Session 1:

100m Load Carry, 20 T Press/Push Ups, 20 Lower Back Raises. As many rounds as possible in 20 minutes.

Conditioning Session 2:

200 Skips, 10 Sandbag Shoulder-to-Shoulder Press, 15 Toes-to-Bar, 20 Box Jumps. 5 rounds.

Workout	Exercise	Weight	Time
Conditioning session 1	100m Load Carry, 20 T Press/Push Ups, 20 Lower Back Raises. As many rounds as possible in 20 minutes.		
Conditioning session 2	200 Skips, 10 Sandbag Shoulder-to-Shoulder Press, 15 Toes-to-Bar, 20 Box Jumps. 5 rounds.		Rounds x

Week 5: Strength

Strength Session 1:

Sandbag Suitcase Deadlift: 5X5
Sandbag Snatch: 4X10
Sandbag Push Jerk: 4X10
T Press/Push Ups: 3 sets to failure
Toes-to-Bar: 3 sets to failure

Strength Session 2:

Sandbag Bear Hug Squat: 5X5
Sandbag Thruster: 5X5
Sandbag Shouldering: 4X10
Hanging Leg Raises: 3 sets to failure
Sandbag Bent Press: 3X5

Week 5: Strength

Workout	Exercise	Reps/Weight	Reps/Weight	Reps/Weight	Reps/Weight	Reps/Weight
Strength session 1	Sandbag Suitcase Deadlift	/	/	/	/	/
	Sandbag Snatch	/	/	/	/	
	Sandbag Push Jerk	/	/	/	/	
	T Press/ Push Up					
	Toes-to-Bar					
Strength session 2	Sandbag Bear Hug Squat	/	/	/	/	/
	Sandbag Thruster	/	/	/	/	/
	Sandbag Shouldering	/	/	/	/	
	Hanging Leg Raises					
	Sandbag Bent Press	/	/	/		

Week 5: Conditioning

Conditioning Session 1:

10 L Pull Ups, 10 Sandbag Clean and Push Jerks, 10 Sandbag Overhead Walking Lunges, 10 Sandbag Bear Hug Squats, 10 Sandbag Snatch. 5 rounds.

Conditioning Session 2:

1000m (1km) run. 10-1 of Sandbag Push Press, Hanging Leg Raises, Sandbag Single Arm Swing.

Workout	Exercise	Weight	Time
Conditioning session 1	10 L Pull Ups, 10 Sandbag Clean and Push Jerks, 10 Sandbag Overhead Walking Lunges, 10 Sandbag Bear Hug Squats, 10 Sandbag Snatch. 5 rounds.		Rounds x
Conditioning session 2	1000m (1km) run. 10-1 of Sandbag Push Press, Hanging Leg Raises, Sandbag Single Arm Swing.		

Week 6: Strength

Strength Session 1:

Sandbag Deadlift: 5X5
Sandbag Clean: 5X5
Sandbag Bent Over Row: 5X5
Sandbag Good Mornings: 4X10
Handstand Press/Push Ups: 5 sets to failure

Strength Session 2:

Sandbag Shoulder Squat: 5X5
Sandbag Floor Press: 5X5
Gorilla Pull Ups: 5 sets to failure
Sandbag Shoulder Get Ups: 4X5
Sandbag Round-the-Worlds: 5X20

Week 6: Strength

Workout	Exercise	Reps/Weight	Reps/Weight	Reps/Weight	Reps/Weight	Reps/Weight
Strength session 1	Sandbag Deadlift	/	/	/	/	/
	Sandbag Clean	/	/	/	/	/
	Sandbag Bent Over Row	/	/	/	/	/
	Sandbag Good Mornings	/	/	/	/	
	Handstand Press/ Push Ups					
Strength session 2	Sandbag Shoulder Squat	/	/	/	/	/
	Sandbag Floor Press	/	/	/	/	/
	Gorilla Pull Ups					
	Sandbag Shoulder Get Ups	/	/	/	/	
	Sandbag Round-the-Worlds	/	/	/	/	/

Week 6: Conditioning

Conditioning Session 1:

Sandbag Hill Sprint (sprint up a 40-60m hill carrying a sandbag). 10 Sandbag Floor Press at the bottom of the hill. As many rounds as possible in 20 minutes.

Conditioning Session 2:

150 Skips, 20 Burpees, 15 High Pulls, 10 Sandbag Thrusters. 5 rounds.

Workout	Exercise	Weight	Time
Conditioning session 1	Sandbag Hill Sprint (sprint up a 40-60m hill carrying a sandbag). 10 Sandbag Floor Press at the bottom of the hill. As many rounds as possible in 20 minutes.		
Conditioning session 2	150 Skips, 20 Burpees, 15 High Pulls, 10 Sandbag Thrusters. 5 rounds.		

Week 7: Strength

Strength Session 1:

Sandbag Suitcase Deadlift: 5X5
Sandbag Snatch: 4X5
Sandbag Push Jerk: 5X5
T Press/Push Ups: 5 sets to failure
Toes-to-Bar: 5 sets to failure

Strength Session 2:

Sandbag Zercher Squats: 5X5
Sandbag Overhead Press: 5X5
Sandbag High Pulls: 5X5
Gorilla Pull Ups: 5 sets to failure
Sandbag Windmills: 5X5

Week 7: Strength

Workout	Exercise	Reps/Weight	Reps/Weight	Reps/Weight	Reps/Weight	Reps/Weight
Strength session 1	Sandbag Suitcase Deadlift	/	/	/	/	/
	Sandbag Snatch	/	/	/	/	
	Sandbag Push Jerk	/	/	/	/	/
	T Press/ Push Up					
	Toes-to-Bar					
Strength session 2	Sandbag Zercher Squats	/	/	/	/	/
	Sandbag Overhead Press	/	/	/	/	/
	Sandbag High Pulls	/	/	/	/	/
	Gorilla Pull Ups					
	Sandbag Windmills	/	/	/	/	/

Week 7: Conditioning

Conditioning Session 1:

5 Gorilla Pull Ups, 10 Handstand Press/Push Ups,15 Sandbag Shoulder Squats. 10 rounds.

Conditioning Session 2:

5 Sandbag Cleans, 5 Sandbag Push Jerks, 5 Sandbag Zercher Squats, 5 Sandbag Good Mornings.

Workout	Exercise	Weight	Time
Conditioning session 1	5 Gorilla Pull Ups, 10 Handstand Press/Push Ups,15 Sandbag Shoulder Squats. 10 rounds.		
Conditioning session 2	5 Sandbag Cleans, 5 Sandbag Push Jerks, 5 Sandbag Zercher Squats, 5 Sandbag Good Mornings.		

Week 8: Strength

Strength Session 1:

Sandbag Deadlift: 5X5
Sandbag Power Cleans: 5X5
Sandbag Bent Over Row: 5X5
Sandbag Good Mornings: 5X5
Sandbag Round-the-Worlds: 5 sets to failure

Strength Session 2:

Sandbag Front Squat: 5X5
Sandbag Floor Press: 5X5
Sandbag High Pulls: 5X5
L Pull Ups: 4 sets to failure
Sandbag Get Ups: 4X5

Week 8: Strength

Workout	Exercise	Reps/ Weight	Reps/ Weight	Reps/ Weight	Reps/ Weight	Reps/ Weight
Strength session 1	Sandbag Deadlift	/	/	/	/	/
	Sandbag Power Cleans	/	/	/	/	/
	Sandbag Bent Over Row	/	/	/	/	/
	Sandbag Good Mornings	/	/	/	/	/
	Sandbag Round-the-Worlds	/	/	/	/	/
Strength session 2	Sandbag Front Squat	/	/	/	/	/
	Sandbag Floor Press	/	/	/	/	/
	Sandbag High Pulls	/	/	/	/	/
	L Pull Ups					
	Sandbag Get Ups	/	/	/	/	

Week 8: Conditioning

Conditioning Session 1:

100m Load Carry, 20 T Press/Push Ups, 20 Lower Back Raises. As many rounds as possible in 20 minutes.

Conditioning Session 2:

200 Skips, 10 Sandbag Shoulder-to-Shoulder Press, 15 Toes-to-Bar, 20 Box Jumps. 5 rounds.

Workout	Exercise	Weight	Time
Conditioning session 1	100m Load Carry, 20 T Press/Push Ups, 20 Lower Back Raises. As many rounds as possible in 20 minutes.		
Conditioning session 2	200 Skips, 10 Sandbag Shoulder-to-Shoulder Press, 15 Toes-to-Bar, 20 Box Jumps. 5 rounds.		Rounds x

Week 9: Strength

Strength Session 1:

Sandbag Suitcase Deadlift: 5X5
Sandbag Snatch: 5X10
Sandbag Push Jerk: 5X10
T Press/Push Ups: 5 sets to failure
Toes-to-Bar: 5 sets to failure

Strength Session 2:

Sandbag Bear Hug Squat: 5X5
Sandbag Thruster: 5X5
Sandbag Shouldering: 5X10
Hanging Leg Raises: 5 sets to failure
Sandbag Bent Press: 5X5

Week 9: Strength

Workout	Exercise	Reps/Weight	Reps/Weight	Reps/Weight	Reps/Weight	Reps/Weight
Strength session 1	Sandbag Suitcase Deadlift	/	/	/	/	/
	Sandbag Snatch	/	/	/	/	/
	Sandbag Push Jerk	/	/	/	/	/
	T Press/ Push Up					
	Toes-to-Bar					
Strength session 2	Sandbag Bear Hug Squat	/	/	/	/	/
	Sandbag Thruster	/	/	/	/	/
	Sandbag Shouldering	/	/	/	/	/
	Hanging Leg Raises					
	Sandbag Bent Press	/	/	/	/	/

Week 9: Conditioning

Conditioning Session 1:

10 L Pull Ups, 10 Sandbag Clean and Push Jerks, 10 Sandbag Overhead Walking Lunges, 10 Sandbag Bear Hug Squats, 10 Sandbag Snatch. 5 rounds.

Conditioning Session 2:

1000m (1km) run. 10-1 of Sandbag Push Press, Hanging Leg Raises, Sandbag Single Arm Swing.

Workout	Exercise	Weight	Time
Conditioning session 1	10 L Pull Ups, 10 Sandbag Clean and Push Jerks, 10 Sandbag Overhead Walking Lunges, 10 Sandbag Bear Hug Squats, 10 Sandbag Snatch. 5 rounds.		Rounds x
Conditioning session 2	1000m (1km) run. 10-1 of Sandbag Push Press, Hanging Leg Raises, Sandbag Single Arm Swing.		

Week 10: Sandbag Challenge!

Do the exercises in the order that they are listed and record your performance. Aim to work as hard as you can and get the best possible score. You should aim to beat your previous best scores for the exercises below.

Take 5 minutes rest between each exercise.

- T Press/Push Ups - perform as many repetitions as possible
- Toes-to-Bar - perform as many repetitions as possible
- L Pull Ups - perform as many repetitions as possible
- Handstand Press/Push Ups - perform as many repetitions as possible

- Sandbag Overhead Walking Lunge - take a moderately heavy sandbag as perform as many repetitions as possible
- Sandbag Clean and Push Jerk - take a moderately heavy sandbag and perform as many repetitions as possible
- Sandbag Bent Press - perform as many repetitions as possible. Repeat with both arms
- Sandbag Shoulder Squat - take a moderately heavy sandbag and perform as many repetitions as possible

- Run 4km - run as fast as possible

Did you improve over the past 10 weeks?

CONGRATULATIONS!

You're through the Advanced Programme!

Your Next Challenge

Congratulations on making it through the Beginner, Intermediate and Advanced sandbag training programmes. You should have seen some serious improvement in strength, conditioning and general health.

The Sandbag Fitness blog has weekly workouts that you can follow and we'd love to have you join in with them. You can add your performance to our comments page and see how you compare with some of our other followers.

Alternatively, you might wish to re-visit the programmes from this guide and try to beat your past performances - this is a great idea too.

However you decide to continue training I hope you've enjoyed this guide.

FAQ

Can I follow Sandbag Fitness and other programmes at the same time? e.g.

- Primal Blueprint Fitness
- Simplefit
- Crossfit
- Wendler 5-3-1
- Starting Strength

Absolutely. We follow many of the same ideas used in these programmes except that we do it with a sandbag. The principles inherent these programmes are strong - we just apply them in a slightly different way. Please do consider though that your results will often be specific to the programme you follow - so if you really want to get good at Barbell lifting then you're going to have to base your programme around that.

Above everything, we aim to show that the sandbag is a viable and accessible alternative to traditional free weights, with plenty of its own merits too.

Do I need to follow any particular dietary approach?

I follow a low Carbohydrate approach with a predominantly unprocessed diet and this suits me very well. For improved energy and body composition I would generally recommend reading the following books:

- The Paleo Solution
- The Primal Blueprint

FAQ

What's really better - a homemade sandbag or a custom made sandbag?

As I said in the Equipment section of this guide, there are advantages for each. With a homemade sandbag you will need to accept that it may break or tear at some stage. Brute Force Sandbags are made to be virtually indestructible and my recommendation is to get yourself one - it will give you many years of training.

What happens when I get to the end of the programmes?

At that stage you would have built a very good level of strength and conditioning with the sandbag. My recommendation would be to then follow the weekly workouts at Sandbag Fitness or, if you don't feel ready, repeat any of the programmes again - ensuring that you focus on improving times and the amount of weight you can lift.

Will I lose weight on this programme?

Weight loss is generally achieved through attention to your diet. This programme is geared towards improving your fitness, strength and conditioning. There is certainly some crossover but I recommend looking at both diet and exercise to get the best results.

FAQ

"I've tried sandbag lifting but I can't lift as much - is that a problem?"

This is common among people who haven't done a lot of sandbag lifting before. You could say that this represents a similar argument to the Leg Press vs. Squat debate. We can all lift more on the leg press but is it meaningful?

Sandbag lifting is tough but I like to see it as a truer representation of my actual strength. The sandbag is a "real world" object - it is rare that you will find a nice handle to grip onto when you have to lift something outside of the gym environment.

In a similar vein, I often speak to people who particularly struggle with getting the sandbag up to chest height so they can press it. But in the real world, if you can't clean it then you can't press it. I view sandbag training in this way too.

To also develop improved Absolute Strength I suggest you include some Barbell work alongside any sandbag training that you do.

FAQ

How much sand will I need and where should I get it from?

It is impossible to work out exactly what you will need as an individual but I would certainly recommend having a range of sandbags - or getting a sandbag that can be easily adjusted. You will need the option of lifting lighter and heavier if you are following the 8 week programme.

The following is a rough starting point for most individuals:

Males:	Light Sandbag	15kg or 33lb
	Medium Sandbag	25kg or 55lb
	Heavy Sandbag	40kg or 88lb
Females:	Light Sandbag	7.5kg or 16.5lb
	Medium Sandbag	15kg or 33lb
	Heavy Sandbag	25kg or 55lb

You can purchase sand from any hardware store at a very low price. You can use any type of sand but you needn't waste your money on fine-filtered sand - the coarse stuff is, in many ways, more practical.

Connect With Us

Watch videos, follow the daily workouts and post your times on the Sandbag Fitness blog.
www.sandbagfitness.blogspot.com

We post all of our workouts on our Facebook page.
www.facebook.com/sandbagfitness

We're always looking to connect with people following the workouts so if you've got pictures of your garage gym or video of you training then we'd love to see them too.
matthewpalfrey@gmail.com

My Youtube channel has some useful instructional video for Sandbag Fitness.
www.youtube.com/user/CoachPalfrey

The Sandbag Fitness Store has a range of sandbag training products and services.
www.sandbagfitnessstore.com

Glossary

Agility

Agility is defined as "the ability to change your body's position efficiently". We use it to describe efficient body movement - with and without the sandbag.

Anyhow Lift

The Anyhow Lift is exactly as the name suggests - you must simply lift the sandbag in the easiest possible manner to whatever location specified (e.g. the chest or overhead)

Barbell

The Barbell is the traditional implement for free weight training. They are, as standard, 7ft bars and weigh 20kg. If you're interested in developing high levels of strength and power then you should also include Barbell training in your programme.

Compound Exercise

A Compound Exercise is one that utilises multiple muscles and joints. These types of exercises have a greater transfer into the majority of "real-life" situations. Sandbag Fitness is based around Compound Exercises.

Conventional/Traditional Free Weights

Conventional Weights, at least in the commercial sense, would be things like Barbells, Dumbbells and Kettlebells.

Glossary

Core Strength/Control

Core Strength refers to your ability to maintain good spinal alignment. It is often, incorrectly, thought of as the Abdominals. When, in fact, in should include all of the musculature of the torso - as they all have an impact on spinal alignment. Core Strength should include activities where you are required to maintain spinal alignment in both static (not moving) and dynamic (moving) positions.

Crunch

The Crunch is an exercise that has largely replaced the Sit Up - predominantly for fears that the Sit Up caused back problems. In reality, the Sit Up just exacerbated pre-existing conditions. The Crunch is considered dysfunctional in comparison to the Sit Up in that it doesn't train the individual to be able to actually "sit up". Excessive use of the Crunch can also cause rounding of the shoulders.

Endurance

The ability to perform a given workload repeatedly without rest.

Filler Bags

The fillable inserts that go inside a Brute Force Sandbag. I sometimes utilise mine for Sandbag Round-the-Worlds - they are not recommended for this though.

Glossary

Functional Training

Overly bastardised Fitness Industry term to describe, predominantly, Stability Training. Commonly used to describe Wobble Boards and Stability Balls. Functional Training should always relate to the individual. So, if you need to be able to lift heavy sacks as part of your daily life then basing your training programme around this would be sensible.

Ground-to-Overhead

Refers to a lift in the "Anyhow" style. You must simply lift the sandbag from the ground to overhead in whatever way you find easiest.

Inverted Row/Australian Pull Ups

Lying underneath a bar of some sort, with your body in a straight line, and pulling yourself up towards the bar. Can also be performed on Gymnastic Rings. This is an easier version of a Pull Up.

Kipping Pull Ups

A style of Pull Ups made popular by Crossfit. It involves aiding the pull by swinging the legs and kicking up into each repetition.

Metabolic Conditioning

Refers to high intensity circuit style training in which there are minimal rest periods. Also known as Met-Con.

Glossary

Neutral spine

The ability to maintain a natural curve in the lower spine.

Pistols

A single-leg squat. Helps to develop balance.

Power

Loosely translated as a "combination of both strength and speed". We use it to describe the ability to move moderate to heavy sandbags at speed.

Repetitions

A repetition is a single performance of an exercise. E.g. One Squat is one repetition of a Squat. Also known as a Rep.

ROM

Refers to Range Of Motion. Can be used to describe the range of motion around a particular joint or, more commonly, the "size" of an exercise - we encourage a full range of motion for all of the exercises listed here. ROM can also be increased E.g. By elevating your body for Press/Push Ups; I use paint cans.

Glossary

Sets

A Set is a collection of consecutive Repetitions. E.g. A Set of 10 Squats is 10 Squats performed in a row without a break.

Strength

Defined as the ability to apply force.

Tornado Ball

A Tornado Ball is traditionally a weighted ball attached to a rope of some type. We make our own using a sandbag and use it to develop rotational power as in the Sandbag Round-the-World.

Copyright

The Complete Guide To Sandbag Training

Images by Alison Crocker

First Edition

Printed in Great Britain
by Amazon.co.uk, Ltd.,
Marston Gate.